CORECTEC'S

COMPREHENSIVE SET OF REVIEW QUESTIONS FOR RADIOGRAPHY

BY
GERALD R. CUMMINGS, B.S.R.T.(R)(QM),M.B.A.
ELIZABETH MEIXNER, R.T.(R)(MR),M.Ed.

Printed in U.S. of America
SIXTH EDITION

TABLE OF CONTENTS:

CHAPTER ONE

RADIATION PROTECTION

- Radiation Detection (62 questions)
- Patient Protection (42 questions)
- Personnel Protection (36 questions)
- Radiation Biology (50 questions)
- Effects of Radiation (40 questions)
- Radiation Regulations (30 questions)

RADIATION DETECTION

1. Which of the following is the unit of absorbed radiation dose?

   A. Rad
   B. Rem
   C. RBE
   D. Roentgen

A

2. Which of the following personnel monitoring devices is capable of providing an immediate reading?

   A. Film badge
   B. Ring badge
   C. Pocket dosimeter
   D. Thermoluminescent dosimeter

C

3. Of the following types of radiation, which one is considered the most ionizing?

   A. Alpha
   B. Beta
   C. Gamma
   D. X Ray

A

4. The Geiger counter is capable of detecting which of the following type(s) of radiation?

   1. X rays
   2. Gamma rays
   3. Beta particles

   A. 1 only
   B. 2 only
   C. 1 & 2 only
   D. 1, 2 & 3

D

5. The time it takes for a radioactive material to have 1/2 of its atoms disintegrate is known as what?

   A. Lethal dose
   B. Half-life
   C. Degree of disintegration
   D. Specific ionization

B

6. While wearing a lead apron, where should the radiation monitor be worn?

   A. On the collar, outside the apron
   B. At the waist, outside the apron
   C. At the waist, under the apron
   D. On the wrist

A

7. Which of the following would be considered natural background radiation?

   1. X rays
   2. Cosmic rays
   3. Alpha particles

   A. 2 only
   B. 3 only
   C. 2 & 3 only
   D. 1, 2 & 3

C

8. Which of the following is a radiation survey instrument?

   A. Gamma camera
   B. Cutie pie
   C. Pocket dosimeter
   D. Thermoluminescent dosimeter

B

9. The reduction of the intensity of radiation as it passes through a material is known as what?

   A. Attenuation
   B. Linear energy coefficient
   C. Linear energy transfer
   D. Absorption

A

10. Which of the following is the least expensive type of radiation monitoring device?

   A. Thermoluminescent dosimeter (TLD)
   B. Optically stimulated luminescence dosimeter (OSL)
   C. Film badge
   D. Pocket dosimeter

C

11. Which of the following is the unit of exposure dose of gamma or x rays?

   A. Rad
   B. Rem
   C. RBE
   D. Roentgen

D

12. Which of the following timers is used to accurately and automatically reproduce radiographic densities?

   A. Mechanical timer
   B. Impulse timer
   C. Electronic timer
   D. Phototimer

D

13. Radiation monitoring instruments depend on which of the following?

1. Space charge
2. Ionization
3. Electrification

A. 1 only
B. 2 only
C. 1 & 2 only
D. 1 & 3 only

B

14. Which of the following radiation monitoring devices is considered to be the most accurate?

A. Film badge
B. Ring badge
C. Optically stimulated luminescence dosimeter (OSL)
D. Thermoluminescent dosimeter (TLD)

C

15. If the exposure rate is 10 R/minute at 40 inches, what will be the rate at 20 inches?

A. 20 R/minute
B. 40 R/minute
C. 60 R/minute
D. 80 R/minute

B

16. Which of the following describes an Alpha particle?

A. Fast neutron
B. 2 protons
C. 2 protons, 2 neutrons
D. Highly energized electron

C

17. The allowable radiation dosage that is assumed to result in an average nominal lifetime risk is known as what?

A. Whole body dose
B. Dose equivalent limits
C. Genetically significant dose
D. Maximum permissible dose

B

18. How many half-value layers are required to reduce a 100 R/minute exposure rate to 25 R/minute?

A. 1
B. 2
C. 4
D. 8

B

19. A piece of paper will provide adequate protection from which of the following types of radiation?

    A. Alpha
    B. Beta
    C. Gamma
    D. X Ray

A

20. Which of the following interactions will occur in the diagnostic x-ray range?

    1. Coherent (classical) scatter
    2. Compton effect
    3. Photoelectric absorption

    A. 1 only
    B. 1 & 2 only
    C. 2 & 3 only
    D. 1, 2 & 3

C

21. Which of the following refers to the measuring of the quantity of an x-ray beam?

    A. Quality control
    B. Quantity control
    C. Beam assurance
    D. Dosimetry

D

22. The becquerel (curie) is a measurement of which of the following?

    A. Number of atoms in an element
    B. Number of gamma rays emitted
    C. Number of disintegrations per second
    D. Number of possible radioisotopes

C

23. Radiation that leaves the tube housing by any means other than through the window is called what?

    A. Primary radiation
    B. Scatter radiation
    C. Leakage radiation
    D. Remnant (exit) radiation

C

24. Which of the following types of radiation is most penetrating?

    A. Alpha
    B. Beta
    C. Gamma
    D. All are equally penetrating

C

25. Which of the following types of radiation is classified as electromagnetic?

1. Alpha
2. Beta
3. Gamma

A. 1 only
B. 2 only
C. 3 only
D. 1 & 2 only

C

26. Radiation that changes direction as it passes through a material is called what?

A. Secondary
B. Scatter
C. Leakage
D. Remnant (exit)

B

27. Which of the following are by-products of photoelectric absorption?

1. Photoelectron
2. Characteristic ray
3. Ionized atom

A. 1 & 2 only
B. 1 & 3 only
C. 2 & 3 only
D. 1, 2 & 3

D

28. The probability of photoelectric absorption occurring increases with an increase in which of the following?

1. kVp
2. Atomic number of material
3. Distance from material

A. 1 only
B. 2 only
C. 3 only
D. 1 & 2 only

B

29. What is the cumulative dose equivalent limits for a 25 year old radiation worker?

A. 50 mSv (5 rem)
B. 100 mSv (10 rem)
C. 250 mSv (25 rem)
D. 350 mSv (35 rem)

C

30. Which of the following is a major disadvantage of a film badge as a radiation monitoring device?

A. Radiation types cannot be determined
B. Immediate readings are not available
C. Must be changed monthly
D. They are grossly inaccurate

B

31. Which of the following refers to the primary beam after it has passed through the beam restricting device?

A. Useful beam
B. Exit beam
C. Secondary beam
D. Stem beam

A

32. Approximately how many rem per image will a female receive to her gonadal area during an IVU examination?

A. .25 rem
B. 1.0 rem
C. 2.5 rem
D. 5.0 rem

A

33. Where should a radiation worker's radiation monitor be located if he is receiving a medical radiographic exam?

A. On the collar of the patient gown
B. Lying on x-ray table - at eye level
C. Lying on x-ray table - waist high
D. Not in the radiographic room

D

34. Which of the following refers to biological dose?

A. Rad
B. Rem
C. RBE
D. Roentgen

C

35. What are the two general types of radiation detection devices?

A. Field survey and personnel monitoring
B. Survey meters and badges
C. Pocket and portable dosimeters
D. Particle and ray detectors

A

36. Which of the following is the unit for measuring the activity of a radionuclide?

    A. Rad
    B. Rem
    C. Curie
    D. Roentgen

C

37. What do the letters "LET" stand for?

    A. Lethal effective tolerance
    B. Lethal exchange table
    C. Linear energy transmutation
    D. Linear energy transfer

D

38. How does the energy of scatter radiation compare to that of the primary beam?

    A. Less energy
    B. More energy
    C. Equal energy
    D. Doubled energy

A

39. How many milliroentgen are in one roentgen?

    A. 10
    B. 100
    C. 1000
    D. 5000

C

40. Which of the following refers to the fact that different types of radiation have different biological effects?

    A. Roentgen
    B. Rad
    C. Rem
    D. RBE

D

41. How often should personnel radiation monitoring devices be changed?

    A. Weekly
    B. Monthly
    C. Quarterly
    D. Yearly

B

42. What is meant by ionizing radiation?

A. Any electromagnetic radiation
B. Any radiation capable of removing an orbital electron
C. Any radiation emitted after ionization
D. Diagnostic x rays

B

43. Which of the following affects the rate of decay of a radioactive material?

A. Pressure
B. Temperature
C. Elevation
D. Nothing can affect the rate of decay

D

44. Which of the following interactions will NOT result in a scatter photon?

A. Photoelectric absorption
B. Compton effect
C. Thompson
D. Coherent (classical)

A

45. Which of the following describes a Beta particle?

A. High speed photon
B. High speed electron
C. High speed proton
D. High speed neutron

B

46. How is the roentgen unit determined?

A. Absorbed dose
B. Ionization in air
C. Half-value layer
D. Compared with rem

B

47. During fluoroscopy, which of the following will produce the greatest amount of scatter radiation?

A. Tube housing
B. Table top
C. Patient
D. Image intensifier

C

48. The roentgen unit only applies to which of the following types of radiation?

A. Alpha
B. Beta
C. X & gamma rays
D. Background

C

49. Why do film badge holders have filters inside?

A. To block alpha particles
B. To block beta particles
C. To prevent backscatter
D. To determine the radiation's energies

D

50. Which of the following filters would produce an x-ray beam with the highest average photon energy?

A. 1 mm Al
B. 2 mm Al
C. 3 mm Al
D. 4 mm Al

D

51. Which of the following x-ray interactions occurs most often with x-ray energies over 100 keV?

A. Coherent (classical) scatter
B. Compton effect
C. Photoelectric absorption
D. Pair production

B

52. Which of the following refers to the amount of ionizing radiation energy transferred by any type of radiation to any target material?

A. RBE
B. Rad
C. Rem
D. Roentgen

B

53. Which of the following statements concerning the roentgen is true?

1. It is measured by ions in air
2. It only measures x and gamma rays
3. Measurement is affected by humidity

A. 1 only
B. 1 & 2 only
C. 1 & 3 only
D. 1, 2 & 3

D

54. The density of a film badge is compared to which of these to determine the exposure to the worker?

A. Density standard
B. National standard
C. Control film badge
D. Fellow technologist's film badge

A

55. The rad, the rem and the roentgen will all be equal when measuring which type of radiation?

A. Alpha
B. Beta
C. X ray
D. Neutrino

C

56. A measure of the number of ion pairs produced in air by a quantity of x rays defines which of these?

A. Rad
B. Rem
C. Joule
D. Roentgen

D

57. The fact that some materials can store energy, then emit light when heated, is the principle that is used for which of these?

A. Ion detector
B. Thermoluminescent dosimeter (TLD)
C. Rate meter
D. Proportional spectrometer

B

58. Which of the following is the quantity of radiation received by radiation workers?

A. Rad
B. Rem
C. RBE
D. Roentgen

B

59. Which of the following measurements is equal to 1 joule per kilogram?

A. Gray
B. Sievert
C. RBE
D. Coulomb/kg

A

60. What do the letters "rem" stand for?

A. Radiation effective measure
B. Rad equivalent man
C. Roentgen energy measurement
D. Radiation energy management

B

61. Which of these is a measure of the rate at which energy is transferred from radiation to soft tissue?

A. Rad
B. Erg
C. LET
D. RBE

C

62. The optically stimulated luminescence (OSL) dosimeter uses which of the following to detect radiation?

A. Aluminum oxide
B. Silver bromide
C. Calcium tungstate
D. Cesium iodide

A

PATIENT PROTECTION

63. What is the primary purpose of beam filtration?

A. Improve radiographic contrast
B. Protect patient from low energy x rays
C. Produce uniform densities on image
D. Increase visibility of detail

B

64. Patient dose during fluoroscopy can be minimized by which of the following?

1. Decrease tube to tower distance
2. Restrict beam size
3. Increase fluoroscopic milliamperage

A. 1 only
B. 2 only
C. 3 only
D. 1 & 3 only

B

65. Which of the following radiographic techniques will provide the least amount of exposure to the patient?

A. 400 mAs, 60 kVp
B. 200 mAs, 70 kVp
C. 100 mAs, 80 kVp
D. 50 mAs, 92 kVp

D

66. What is the dose equivalent limits for a non-radiation worker?

A. 2.5 mSv (.25 rem)/year
B. 5.0 mSv (0.5 rem)/year
C. 12 mSv (1.2 rem)/year
D. 25 mSv (2.5 rem)/year

B

67. Which of the following will NOT have an effect on patient dose?

A. Filtration
B. SID
C. Focal spot size
D. kVp

C

68. The function of a beam filter is to remove which of the following from the x-ray beam?

A. Secondary radiation
B. Scatter radiation
C. Low energy radiation
D. High energy radiation

C

69. When should gonadal shielding be used on a patient?

1. If the patient is of a reproductive age or younger
2. If the shield will not interfere with the exam
3. If the gonads lie in or near the primary beam

A. 1 & 2 only
B. 1 & 3 only
C. 2 & 3 only
D. 1, 2 & 3

D

70. Which of the following will NOT reduce the amount of exposure to the patient?

A. Higher grid ratio
B. Proper collimation
C. Beam filtration
D. Use of intensifying screens

A

71. Which of the following are features of fluoroscopic equipment designed to reduce unnecessary radiation to the patient?

1. Collimation
2. Protective lead curtain
3. Deadman switch

A. 1 only
B. 2 only
C. 1 & 2 only
D. 1 & 3 only

D

72. Which of the following radiographic procedures will require gonadal shielding?

A. Chest
B. Knee
C. Unilateral hip
D. Skull series

C

73. Which type of gonadal shielding could be used for a patient having an exam requiring a sterile field?

A. Lead sheet
B. Lead apron
C. Shadow shield
D. Pseudo shield

C

74. The 10-day rule applies to which of the following patient types?

A. Pediatric patients
B. Geriatric patients
C. Females of a reproductive age
D. Males of a reproductive age

C

75. Which of the following will reduce exposure to the patient as well as improve radiographic contrast?

1. Beam restriction
2. Increase screen speed
3. Highest recommended developer temp.

A. 1 & 2 only
B. 1 & 3 only
C. 2 & 3 only
D. 1, 2 & 3

B

76. According to the 10-day rule, when is the safest time to radiograph a female?

    A. 10 days prior to the menstrual cycle
    B. 10 days after the menstrual cycle
    C. 10 days during the menstrual cycle
    D. 10 days after the onset of the menstrual cycle

D

77. Which of the following is NOT an important factor when attempting to reduce patient exposure?

    A. Use highest possible mAs
    B. Use close collimation
    C. Use gonadal shielding
    D. Use well calibrated equipment

A

78. Which of the following examinations would NOT allow male gonadal shielding?

    A. Intravenous urogram
    B. Pelvis examination
    C. Knee arthrogram
    D. Voiding cystourethrogram

D

79. A .5 mm lead gonadal shield will reduce female gonadal exposure by approximately what percentage?

    A. 25%
    B. 50%
    C. 75%
    D. 99%

C

80. The dose rate at the table top during fluoroscopy cannot exceed _____ R per minute.

    A. 2
    B. 5
    C. 7
    D. 10

D

81. Which of the following situations would cause the greatest skin dose to a patient?

    A. Short SID
    B. Long SID
    C. Small focal spot size
    D. Highest practical kilovoltage

A

82. The source-to-skin distance for stationary fluoroscopy must NOT be less than which of the following?

A. 5"
B. 15"
C. 20"
D. 40"

B

83. When using mobile radiographic equipment, the source-to-skin distance cannot be less than what?

A. 12"
B. 24"
C. 36"
D. 48"

A

84. A fetus is most vulnerable to radiation during which of the following time periods?

A. First trimester
B. Second trimester
C. Third trimester
D. Fourth trimester

A

85. Which of the following are things a radiographer should do in order to avoid unnecessary patient exposure?

1. Avoid retaking radiographs
2. Use high speed screens
3. Keep equipment in good working order

A. 1 & 2 only
B. 1 & 3 only
C. 2 & 3 only
D. 1, 2 & 3

D

86. What is the name of the filtration that is a permanent part of the x-ray tube head?

A. Added filtration
B. Inherent filtration
C. Compensating filtration
D. Stem filtration

B

87. Which of the following types of beam restricting devices is considered the best at reducing patient exposure?

A. Cone
B. Diaphragm
C. Collimator
D. Extension cylinder

D

88. How will beam filtration effect the primary beam?

A. Make it more homogeneous
B. Make it more heterogeneous
C. Make it less penetrating
D. Reduce its quality

A

89. To prevent leakage radiation from exposing the patient, an x-ray tube must have how much protective lead?

A. 1.5 mm
B. 2.5 mm
C. 3.5 mm
D. 4.5 mm

A

90. When using over 70 kVp, the total beam filtration must be how much?

A. 1.5 mm Al
B. 2.5 mm Al
C. 3.5 mm Al
D. 4.5 mm Al

B

91. Which of the following effects will result from precise collimation?

1. Less biological tissue is exposed
2. Less scatter radiation is produced
3. Radiographic quality is improved

A. 1 & 2 only
B. 1 & 3 only
C. 2 & 3 only
D. 1, 2 & 3

D

92. How can a fast film-screen combination reduce patient exposure?

A. Requires less kVp
B. Allows for smaller focal spot size
C. Allows for a reduction in mAs
D. Eliminates the need for a grid

C

93. What is the dose equivalent limits for a pregnant female patient?

A. 1 mSv (0.1 rem)
B. 5 mSv (0.5 rem)
C. 15 mSv (1.5 rem)
D. 50 mSv (5.0 rem)

B

94. Which of the following has the greatest effect on the amount of radiation exposure to the patient?

A. Focal spot size
B. SID
C. Size of exposed area
D. Type of grid (linear or cross-hatch)

C

95. Which of the following are disadvantages of using a flat piece of lead for gonadal shielding?

1. Cannot be used for erect views
2. Difficult to keep in place
3. Is not very useful for fluoroscopy

A. 1 & 2 only
B. 1 & 3 only
C. 2 & 3 only
D. 1, 2 & 3

D

96. Which of the following types of equipment could have a great effect on reducing population exposure?

A. Fluoroscopic devices
B. Tomographic machines
C. Automatic exposure control (AEC)
D. Computerized tomography equipment

C

97. Which of the following methods is used to determine if an x-ray tube has adequate filtration?

A. Read tube specifications
B. Physical examination of tube
C. Visual inspection of tube
D. Half-value layer (HVL) measurement

D

98. If 2 mm Al is added to an x-ray beam that has a HVL of 2 mm Al, how much will the exposure be reduced?

A. 25%
B. 50%
C. 75%
D. 95%

B

99. What percentage of the total amount of radiation to the general public is due to medical and dental x rays?

A. 50%
B. 65%
C. 80%
D. 90%

A

100. Which of the following is a means of expressing the dose a patient has received from a radiographic examination?

1. Skin dose
2. Organ dose
3. Whole body dose

A. 1 only
B. 3 only
C. 2 & 3 only
D. 1, 2 & 3

D

101. Which of the following factors will affect the quantity as well as the quality of the x-ray beam?

1. kVp
2. HVL
3. SID

A. 1 only
B. 2 only
C. 2 & 3 only
D. 1, 2 & 3

D

102. Which of the following are reasons for using beam restricting devices?

1. Reduce scatter radiation
2. Reduce patient exposure
3. Improve radiographic contrast

A. 1 & 2 only
B. 1 & 3 only
C. 2 & 3 only
D. 1, 2 & 3

D

103. The quality of an x-ray beam can be measured by which of the following methods?

1. Rate meter
2. Sensitometry
3. Half-value layer

A. 1 only
B. 2 only
C. 3 only
D. 2 & 3 only

C

104. Which of the following could result from excessive radiation exposure to a fetus during the first trimester?

1. Prenatal death
2. Neonatal death
3. Congenital abnormalities

A. 1 only
B. 2 only
C. 3 only
D. 1, 2 & 3

D

PERSONNEL PROTECTION

105. How far must a radiographer stand back during a mobile radiographic exposure?

A. 1 meter
B. 2 meters
C. 3 meters
D. 4 meters

B

106. Personnel monitoring devices are used for which of the following reasons?

1. Because it is a requirement
2. To assure workers receive less than the dose equivalent limit
3. To check radiation safety practices

A. 1 & 2 only
B. 1 & 3 only
C. 2 & 3 only
D. 1, 2 & 3

D

107. Which of the following is the best protection from radiation?

A. Distance
B. Lead glass
C. Lead shield
D. Lead apron

A

108. What is the dose equivalent limits for the hands of a technologist?

A. 50 mSv (5 rem)/year
B. 250 mSv (25 rem)/year
C. 500 mSv (50 rem)/year
D. 750 mSv (75 rem)/year

C

109. What is the dose equivalent limits for the whole body of a radiation worker?

A. 50 mSv (5 rem)/year
B. 250 mSv (25 rem)/year
C. 500 mSv (50 rem)/year
D. 750 mSv (75 rem)/year

A

110. Personnel monitoring is required when there is any likelihood that an individual will receive more than _____ the dose equivalent limits.

A. 1/2
B. 1/6
C. 1/10
D. 1/24

C

111. Which of the following is a primary factor in protecting radiographers from scatter radiation?

A. Increase kVp
B. Reduce focal spot size
C. Use some type of lead shielding
D. Reduce screen speed

C

112. Radiation workers are monitored for radiation exposure by which of the following means?

A. Chest X-ray
B. Radiation monitor
C. Complete blood count (CBC)
D. Gamma camera

B

113. What must the lead equivalency be for a lead apron?

A. .25 mm Pb
B. .50 mm Pb
C. 2.5 mm Pb
D. 5.0 mm Pb

B

114. Where should a radiation monitor be worn to assure that a technologist is NOT receiving too much radiation?

A. On the collar
B. At the waist
C. On the finger
D. In a pocket

A

115. Which of the following individuals should be asked to help hold an uncooperative child?

A. Student
B. Transporter
C. Technologist
D. Parent

D

116. Which of the following is a primary factor in protecting radiographers from scatter radiation?

A. Increase kVp
B. Reduce focal spot size
C. Eliminate the use of grids
D. Increase distance from patient

D

117. How much is radiation exposure reduced if the distance between the patient and technologist is doubled?

A. 2 times less
B. 4 times less
C. 6 times less
D. 8 times less

B

118. Which of the following definitions describes dose equivalent limits?

A. The maximum dose a body can tolerate
B. A dose that is not expected to produce significant effects
C. The dose a worker will receive/year
D. The maximum dose a radiation monitor records

B

119. What is the dose equivalent limits a radiography student may receive in one year if he/she is under 18 years old?

A. 1 mSv (.1 rem)
B. 5 mSv (.5 rem)
C. 10 mSv (1 rem)
D. 50 mSv (5 rem)

A

120. To reduce the amount of scatter radiation, which of the following should be done by the radiographer?

1. Increase kVp and reduce mAs
2. Utilize precise collimation
3. Increase the OID

A. 1 only
B. 2 only
C. 1 and 3 only
D. 1, 2 & 3

B

121. What is the dose equivalent limits to the fetus of a pregnant radiologic technologist?

A. .1 mSv/month
B. .5 mSv/month
C. 1.0 mSv/month
D. 5.0 mSv/month

B

122. How thick must the lead be in a primary barrier of a radiographic room?

A. 1/32"
B. 1/16"
C. 1/8"
D. 1/2"

B

123. The lead equivalency for a pair of protective gloves must be at least how much?

A. .25 mm
B. .50 mm
C. .75 mm
D. 1.5 mm

A

124. During fluoroscopy, where is an acceptable position for the radiographer to stand?

A. In the room, next to the patient
B. In the room, next to the radiologist
C. In the room, as far from the patient as practical
D. Holding the patient

C

125. Which of the following materials is the most effective as a protective barrier?

A. Lead
B. Lead glass
C. Copper
D. Aluminum

A

126. What is the dose equivalent limits a radiation worker can receive in any one quarter (13 weeks) of a year?

A. 10 mSv (1 rem)
B. 30 mSv (3 rem)
C. 50 mSv (5 rem)
D. 70 mSv (7 rem)

B

127. Primary radiation barriers in walls must be how high?

A. 5 feet
B. 7 feet
C. 9 feet
D. 11 feet

B

128. Which of the following describes a primary protective barrier?

1. A lead apron
2. A barrier to absorb scatter radiation
3. A barrier to absorb primary radiation

A. 1 only
B. 3 only
C. 2 & 3 only
D. 1, 2 & 3

B

129. The fact that distance is the best protection against radiation is proven by which of these laws?

A. Ohm's law
B. Inverse square law
C. Coulomb's law
D. Law of conservation of energy

B

130. Mobile protective barriers should NOT be used when making exposures above what kilovoltage?

A. 70 kVp
B. 90 kVp
C. 110 kVp
D. 140 kVp

B

131. When referring to a whole body dose, which of the following is NOT included?

A. Eyes and neck
B. Hands and feet
C. Reproductive organs
D. Blood forming organs

B

132. How many times should radiation scatter before reaching the control booth or a mobile protective barrier?

A. One time
B. Two times
C. Three times
D. Four times

B

133. Which of the following will reduce radiation exposure to personnel?

1. Reduce time of exposure
2. Increase distance from source of radiation
3. Insert shielding between source of radiation and personnel

A. 1 only
B. 2 only
C. 2 & 3 only
D. 1, 2 & 3

D

134. A secondary barrier protects the technologist from which of the following types of radiation?

1. Stem radiation
2. Primary radiation
3. Scatter radiation

A. 2 only
B. 3 only
C. 2 & 3 only
D. 1, 2 & 3

B

135. Which of the following characteristics makes lead such an excellent protective barrier?

1. High density
2. High atomic number
3. High absorption coefficient

A. 1 only
B. 1 & 3 only
C. 2 & 3 only
D. 1, 2 & 3

D

136. What percentage of the primary exposure to the patient will reach a radiographer standing 1 meter away?

A. .1%
B. .5%
C. 2.5%
D. 5.0%

A

137. If an exposure of 16 mR is recorded at 1 meter, what would the exposure rate be at 4 meters?

A. 1 mR
B. 2 mR
C. 4 mR
D. 8 mR

A

138. A radiographer will receive most of his/her occupational exposure from which of these types of radiation?

A. Primary radiation
B. Scatter radiation
C. Remnant (exit) radiation
D. Gamma radiation

B

139. What is the exposure rate if 75 mAs results in an exposure of 600 mR?

A. 6 mR/mAs
B. 8 mR/mAs
C. 60 mR/mAs
D. 80 mR/mAs

B

140. Which of the following would never be considered as a primary barrier in normal diagnostic radiography?

A. A wall
B. The floor
C. The ceiling
D. A mobile shield

C

RADIATION BIOLOGY

141. Human cells are divided into two classifications. They are genetic cells and _____ cells.

A. Organic
B. Benign
C. Somatic
D. Reproductive

C

142. What is the process of cell division of somatic cells called?

A. Meiosis
B. Mitosis
C. Synthesis
D. Multiplication

B

143. Which of the following stages of cell division is considered to be the most radiosensitive?

A. Prophase
B. Anaphase
C. Telophase
D. Metaphase

D

144. The "Direct Hit" theory of cell irradiation can be described by which of the following statements?

A. The DNA molecule is struck
B. The cell nucleus is struck
C. The cell cytoplasm is struck
D. The cell is ionized

A

145. Which of the following mature cells would be least sensitive to radiation?

A. Muscle cells
B. Nerve cells
C. Red blood cells
D. White blood cells

B

146. Which of the following is NOT part of the genetic code that helps compose a DNA molecule?

A. Adenine
B. Cytosine
C. Thymine
D. Urine

D

147. The amount of ionization that occurs when radiation passes through tissue depends on which of the following?

1. The type of radiation
2. The size of the particle
3. The charge on the particle

A. 1 only
B. 1 & 3 only
C. 2 & 3 only
D. 1, 2 & 3

D

148. Which of the following is the most sensitive to radiation?

A. Lymphoid tissue
B. Epithelial tissue
C. Connective tissue
D. Muscle tissue

A

149. Which of the following would describe the shape of a DNA molecule?

A. Elliptical
B. Hypocycloidal
C. Double helix
D. Circular

C

150. Which of the following is a type of damage that can occur to a DNA molecule when exposed to radiation?

1. Change in the genetic code
2. Breakage of the chromosome
3. Breakage of the DNA molecule

A. 1 only
B. 3 only
C. 1 & 3 only
D. 1, 2 & 3

D

151. Where do the metabolic functions of a cell take place?

A. Nucleus
B. Chromosomes
C. Cytoplasm
D. DNA molecule

C

152. How many matched pairs of chromosomes does a human somatic cell contain?

A. 6
B. 13
C. 23
D. 46

C

153. What is the name of the stage of cell division that is commonly referred to as the resting stage?

A. Anaphase
B. Interphase
C. Metaphase
D. Telophase

B

154. An alteration in the sequence of bases in a DNA molecule will result in which of the following?

A. A mutation
B. A duplication
C. A replication
D. A chromatin

A

155. Which of the following are considered the building blocks in the synthesizing of proteins?

A. Genes
B. RNA molecules
C. Chromosomes
D. Amino acids

D

156. Where would the majority of RNA molecules be found in a human cell?

A. Cytoplasm
B. DNA molecule
C. Nucleolus
D. Chromosome

C

157. The somatic effects of radiation refer to which of the following?

A. Exposure to the trunk
B. Exposure to the reproductive organs
C. Exposure to the body tissues
D. Exposure to the nervous system

C

158. Which of the following are considered extremely sensitive to radiation?

1. Gonads
2. Lens of the eye
3. Blood forming organs

A. 1 only
B. 1 & 3 only
C. 2 & 3 only
D. 1, 2 & 3

B

159. The small segments of the DNA molecule that determine the characteristics of each cell are called what?

A. Genes
B. Centrioles
C. Purines
D. Spindle fibers

A

160. Which of the following is the most common result of cell irradiation?

A. Cell death
B. Sterilization
C. Mutation
D. Uncontrolled growth

B

161. Which of the following types of blood cells is the most sensitive to radiation?

A. Lymphocytes
B. Granulocytes
C. Thrombocytes
D. Erythrocytes

A

162. The information that cells require for metabolism is coded in which of the following?

A. Cytoplasm
B. Spindle fibers
C. RNA molecule
D. DNA molecule

D

163. The radiation interaction with tissue that causes most of the cellular damage is which of the following?

A. Excitation
B. Ionization
C. Classical scattering
D. Thompson scattering

B

164. What do the letters "DNA" stand for?

A. Direct nuclear action
B. Deuteron nucleus activity
C. Deoxyribonucleic acid
D. Deoxyribose neutral acid

C

165. Which of the following are the two bases that are the building blocks of both types of nucleic acids?

A. Purines and pyrimidines
B. Adenine and thymine
C. Adenine and quanine
D. Ribose and deoxyribose

A

166. Which of the following pyrimidines will always pair with the purine - adenine?

A. Cytosine
B. Thymine
C. Uracil
D. Quanine

B

167. Which of the following is NOT a stage of somatic cell division?

A. Prophase
B. Metaphase
C. Nanophase
D. Telophase

C

168. How will oxygen retention effect the radiosensitivity of a cell?

A. Radiosensitivity will increase
B. Radiosensitivity will decrease
C. Radiosensitivity will be eliminated
D. Radiosensitivity will not be effected

A

169. Which of the following types of tissue will absorb the most radiation?

A. Air sacs
B. Bone
C. Muscle
D. Soft tissue

B

170. Irradiation of which of the following anatomical areas will affect the production of white blood cells?

A. Lungs
B. Liver
C. Pancreas
D. Bone marrow

D

171. Which of the following describes an atom that has lost one or more of its electrons?

A. Ion
B. Nuclide
C. Isotope
D. Unstable

A

172. Ionization can result from which of the following interactions of radiation with tissue?

1. Photoelectric absorption
2. Compton effect
3. Coherent (classical) scatter

A. 1 only
B. 1 & 2 only
C. 2 & 3 only
D. 1, 2 & 3

B

173. Which of the following interactions of radiation with tissue results in the complete absorption of the photon?

1. Photoelectric absorption
2. Compton effect
3. Coherent (classical) scatter

A. 1 only
B. 1 & 2 only
C. 1 & 3 only
D. 1, 2 & 3

A

174. A chromosome that has been damaged by radiation may cause which of the following?

1. A mutation
2. Cell death
3. Sterilization

A. 1 only
B. 2 only
C. 2 & 3 only
D. 1, 2 & 3

D

175. What is the molecule called that has one or more unpaired electrons and is unusually chemically reactive?

A. Ion
B. Mutation
C. Free radical
D. Excited molecule

C

176. Which of the following is considered the unit of heredity?

A. The cell
B. The gene
C. The chromosome
D. The DNA molecule

B

177. Gross structural changes that arise when radiation breaks a chromosome may be referred to as what?

1. Aberrations
2. Anomalies
3. Lesions

A. 1 & 2 only
B. 1 & 3 only
C. 2 & 3 only
D. 1, 2 & 3

D

178. During mitosis, each chromosome splits in half. What are the two halves called?

A. Chromatids
B. Fragments
C. Centromeres
D. Spindle fibers

A

179. The messenger RNA carries information to which of the following in order to synthesize proteins?

A. DNA molecule
B. Transfer RNA molecule
C. Chromosome
D. Ribosome

D

180. Transfer RNA carries which of the following to the polysome in order to synthesize a protein?

A. Amino acids
B. Polypeptides
C. Anticodons
D. Chromosomes

A

181. Where will most of a cell's genetic information be found?

A. Nucleus
B. Nucleolus
C. Cytoplasm
D. Daughter cell

A

182. What is the process of cell division of the reproductive (genetic) cells called?

A. Meiosis
B. Mitosis
C. Synthesis
D. Multiplication

A

183. Which of the following is the major function of the process of meiosis?

A. Synthesize physical characteristics
B. Reduce number of chromosomes by half
C. Increase the number of germ cells
D. Synthesize proteins

B

184. Which of the following refers to the single set of chromosomes in a genetic cell?

A. Diploid number
B. Triploid number
C. Haploid number
D. Semiloid number

C

185. What do the letters "RBE" stand for?

A. Relative biologic effectiveness
B. Radiosensitive biologic effect
C. Radioactive biological energy
D. Radiation bypass effect

A

186. Of the following blood cell producing organs, which are considered radiosensitive?

1. Spleen
2. Bone marrow
3. Lymphatic nodes

A. 1 & 2 only
B. 1 & 3 only
C. 2 & 3 only
D. 1, 2 & 3

D

187. Which of the following is a correct statement concerning a DNA molecule?

1. It is classified as a nucleic acid
2. It is described as a macromolecule
3. It contains five-carbon sugars

A. 1 only
B. 2 only
C. 2 & 3 only
D. 1, 2 & 3

D

188. The probability of radiation interacting with matter depends on which of the following?

1. The charge of the radiation
2. The size of the radiation
3. The energy of the radiation

A. 1 only
B. 3 only
C. 1 & 3 only
D. 1, 2 & 3

D

189. Which of the following is NOT a function of a DNA molecule?

A. It carries the genetic code
B. It duplicates exact copies of itself
C. It synthesizes proteins
D. It divides during mitosis

C

190. Which of the following is a measure of the rate of energy loss along the track of an ionizing particle?

A. Scintillation counter
B. Linear energy transfer
C. Linear attenuation coefficient
D. Ionization

B

EFFECTS OF RADIATION

191. Which of the following are possible results from the exposure to radiation?

1. Changes in the DNA molecule
2. Sterilization of the cell
3. Death of the cell

A. 1 only
B. 2 only
C. 1 & 3 only
D. 1, 2 & 3

D

192. How can radiation damage to the DNA molecule of a genetic cell affect the future generations of an individual?

A. Mutations may occur
B. Offspring may be radioactive
C. Offspring may be immune to radiation
D. Radiation cannot affect offspring

A

193. Whole body radiation, delivered in a period of seconds to minutes, produces a clinical pattern known as what?

A. Mortality irradiation
B. Cumulative exposure
C. Whole body dose
D. Acute radiation syndrome

D

194. The dose-response curve below could be defined by which of the following?

A. Linear, threshold
B. Linear, non-threshold
C. Non-linear, threshold
D. Non-linear, non-threshold

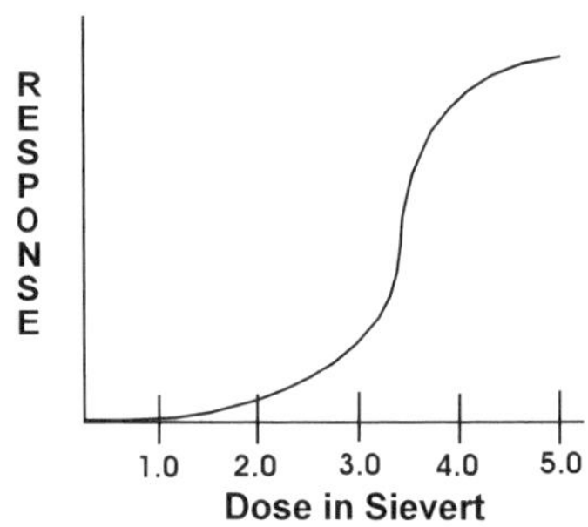

C

195. The dose-response curve above could represent which of the following?

A. Diagnostic x rays
B. Acute radiation syndrome
C. Alpha particles
D. Protein synthesis

B

196. What does lethal dose 50/30 mean?

A. 30 people out of 50 will die
B. 50 people will die within 30 minutes
C. 30 rem will kill half of the group
D. 50% of the group dies within 30 days

D

197. What do the letters "GSD" stand for?

A. Gonadal safe dose
B. Genetically significant dose
C. Genetic-somatic dose
D. General somatic dose

B

198. What does genetically significant dose mean?

A. Dose that will cause damage
B. Dose that will cause genetic damage
C. Dose that will cause a mutation
D. Estimated dose received by the population

D

199. Radiation damage depends on which of the following?

1. Absorbed dose
2. Type of radiation
3. Size of area exposed

A. 1 only
B. 2 only
C. 3 only
D. 1, 2 & 3

D

200. What is the minimum level of radiation exposure below which no genetic or somatic damage occurs?

A. 5 R
B. 10 R
C. 15 R
D. No minimum level is known

D

201. A fluoroscopic procedure performed on a pregnant female could result in which of the following?

1. Stillbirth
2. Miscarriage
3. Congenital anomalies

A. 2 only
B. 1 & 2 only
C. 2 & 3 only
D. 1, 2 & 3

D

202. Radiation is said to be carcinogenic. What does carcinogenic mean?

A. A cancer producing substance
B. Causes genetic changes
C. The ability to destroy cancer
D. Causes cell death

A

203. How can radiation induce cancer in a person?

A. It can alter a cells function
B. A mutation can increase cell growth
C. It can cause cell death
D. Radiation destroys the immune system

B

204. How much radiation exposure does it take to have a lethal dose where 50% of the humans would die within 60 days?

A. 100 to 200 R
B. 200 to 300 R
C. 300 to 400 R
D. 400 to 500 R

C

205. Which of the following would NOT occur from a significant exposure to radiation?

A. Blood disorders
B. Malignant growths develop
C. Cataract formation
D. Immunity to radiation damage

D

206. When radiation exposure causes hematopoietic death, what is the main reason why the person died?

A. Hemorrhage
B. Respiratory distress
C. Immune system is destroyed
D. Heart failure

C

207. The greatest radiation hazard to a fetus occurs during which of the following time periods?

A. First trimester
B. Second trimester
C. Third trimester
D. Fourth trimester

A

208. During a radiographic examination, which of the following would produce the greatest skin dose?

A. High kilovoltage technique
B. Low milliamperage technique
C. Long SID
D. Short SID

D

209. A reddening of the skin due to radiation damage is called what?

A. Emesis
B. Erythema
C. Euploidy
D. Epidermal destruction

B

210. Which of the following are possible long-term somatic effects of ionizing radiation?

1. Life-span shortening
2. Malignant neoplasm
3. Blood deficiencies

A. 1 & 2 only
B. 1 & 3 only
C. 2 & 3 only
D. 1, 2 & 3

D

211. If a human is exposed to radiation levels in the 100 to 200 R range, which of the following is expected?

A. No clinical effects
B. Slight reduction in lymphocytes
C. Complete recovery in 90 days
D. Death within 30 days

C

212. Which statement is true concerning the effects of radiation exposure?

A. No effects occur at low rem levels
B. Damage is not passed on to offspring
C. The body can repair most damage
D. Mutations only occur at high exposure

C

213. Which of the following types of radiation can cause ionization, and therefore biological damage?

1. X rays
2. Infra red
3. Microwaves

A. 1 only
B. 1 & 3 only
C. 2 & 3 only
D. 1, 2 & 3

A

214. Radiation exposure has been linked as a cause of which of the following malignant diseases?

1. Leukemia
2. Skin cancer
3. Thyroid cancer

A. 1 only
B. 2 only
C. 1 & 2 only
D. 1, 2 & 3

D

215. A person exhibiting radiation sickness would have which of the following symptoms?

1. Nausea
2. Diarrhea
3. Loss of appetite

A. 1 only
B. 3 only
C. 1 & 2 only
D. 1, 2 & 3

D

216. Why is radiation exposure to the gonads such a critical concern?

1. The person may become sterile
2. Mutations in offspring may result
3. Gonadal cancer may develop

A. 1 only
B. 2 only
C. 2 & 3 only
D. 1, 2 & 3

B

217. What is the amount of radiation necessary to produce a noticeable skin reaction called?

A. Soft dose
B. Low energy dose
C. Erythema dose
D. Isodose

C

218. Somatic effects of radiation relate to which of the following?

A. The fetus
B. The newborn
C. Future generations
D. The exposed individual

D

219. Which of the following determines what the final effect from radiation will be?

1. Type of radiation
2. Type of tissue
3. Energy of radiation

A. 1 only
B. 3 only
C. 2 & 3 only
D. 1, 2 & 3

D

220. What is the most radiosensitive area of the eye?

A. Iris
B. Lens
C. Cornea
D. Retina

B

221. Which of the following individuals should the radiographer be concerned about when using x rays?

A. A child
B. An adult
C. A radiation worker
D. All of the above need consideration

D

222. How has data been collected for the study of the effects of radiation exposure?

1. Therapy patients
2. Radiation workers
3. Atomic bomb survivors

A. 1 only
B. 3 only
C. 2 & 3 only
D. 1, 2 & 3

D

223. 50% of the radiation exposure to the general population comes from which of the following sources?

A. Nuclear power plants
B. Atomic weapons testing
C. Background radiation
D. Medical and dental radiographs

D

224. Which of these situations will cause the greatest effect from radiation exposure?

A. Small dose over a long time period
B. Large dose over a short time period
C. Small dose over a short time period
D. Large dose over a long time period

B

225. Which of the following cells would be affected by a relatively small amount of radiation exposure?

A. Muscle
B. Nerve
C. Leukocyte
D. Liver

C

226. Which of the following organs is considered radiosensitive?

A. Liver
B. Spleen
C. Gonads
D. Thyroid

C

227. Early radiation therapy treatments for acne, tonsillitis, etc. has resulted in some cases of what?

A. Death
B. Thyroid cancer
C. Brain damage
D. Pineal calcification

B

228. What would be the probable result of any major radiation exposure during the first few days of pregnancy?

A. Prenatal death
B. Postnatal death
C. A child with genetic deficiencies
D. A normal birth and infant

A

229. The dose-response curve below could be defined by which of the following?

A. Linear, threshold
B. Linear, non-threshold
C. Non-linear, threshold
D. Non-linear, non-threshold

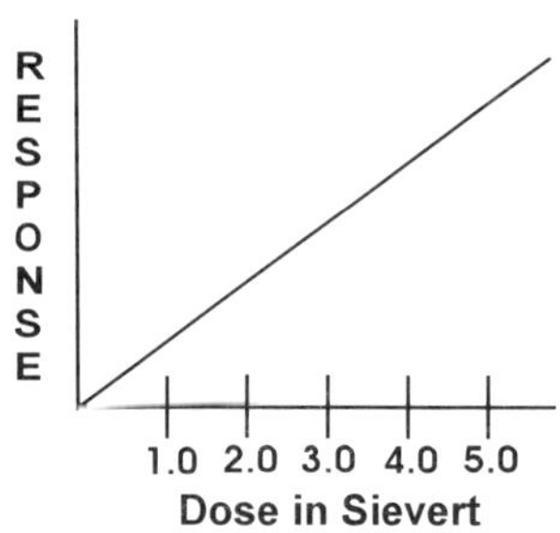

B

230. The dose-response curve above could represent which of the following?

A. Diagnostic x rays
B. Alpha particles
C. Acute radiation syndrome
D. Any electromagnetic radiation

A

RADIATION REGULATIONS

231. Which of the following publications recommends limits of exposure to ionizing radiation?

A. NCRP Report #100
B. NCRP Report #102
C. NCRP Report #105
D. NCRP Report #116

D

232. What is the function of the National Council on Radiation Protection and Measurement?

A. Set standards for using radiation
B. Educate the public about radiation
C. Educate radiation workers
D. Keep records on radiation hazards

A

233. The dose equivalent limits for radiation workers is based on the radiation received from what sources?

A. Background radiation
B. Medical and dental radiography
C. Occupational exposure
D. Radiation fallout

C

234. Standards state that the exposure in air from fluoroscopic equipment shall NOT exceed how many Coulomb/kg/minute?

A. 1.29×10^{-3} Coulomb/kg (5 R)
B. 2.58×10^{-3} Coulomb/kg (10 R)
C. 3.87×10^{-3} Coulomb/kg (15 R)
D. 5.16×10^{-3} Coulomb/kg (20 R)

B

235. The field positioning light and the actual radiation field cannot vary by more than what percentage of the SID?

A. +/- 2%
B. +/- 5%
C. +/-10%
D. +/ 20%

A

236. Which of the following are NOT required on newly manufactured radiographic equipment?

1. Automatic exposure control (AEC)
2. Computerized technique selections
3. Automatic collimators

A. 1 only
B. 2 only
C. 3 only
D. 1, 2 & 3

D

237. Which of the following signals is needed to indicate that a radiation exposure has been made?

A. Laser light
B. Ultraviolet light
C. High frequency sound wave
D. Audible sound and visible light

D

238. Which of the following devices alerts the radiologist that 5 minutes of fluoroscopy has elapsed?

A. Phototimer
B. Cumulative timer
C. Synchronous timer
D. Mechanical timer

B

239. When using over 70 kVp, the total filtration in the primary beam must be at least how much?

A. 1.0 mm Al
B. 2.0 mm Al
C. 2.5 mm Al
D. 3.5 mm Al

C

240. Personnel monitoring shall be performed if there is a possibility of exceeding how many sievert (rem) per year?

A. 2.5 mSv (0.25 rem)
B. 5.0 mSv (0.50 rem)
C. 12.5 mSv (1.25 rem)
D. 25.0 mSv (2.50 rem)

B

241. Leakage radiation from the x-ray tube cannot exceed which of the following at a distance of one meter?

A. 6.45×10^{-6} Coulomb/kg/hr (25 mR/hr)
B. 1.29×10^{-5} Coulomb/kg/hr (50 mR/hr)
C. 1.94×10^{-5} Coulomb/kg/hr (75 mR/hr)
D. 2.58×10^{-5} Coulomb/kg/hr (100 mR/hr)

D

242. What is the dose equivalent limits that the hands and feet may receive?

A. 200 mSv (20 rem)
B. 300 mSv (30 rem)
C. 400 mSv (40 rem)
D. 500 mSv (50 rem)

D

243. Which of the following relates to the dose equivalent limits for a non-radiation worker?

A. 1/10 that of a radiation worker
B. 1/2 that of a radiation worker
C. The same as a radiation worker
D. Twice that of a radiation worker

A

244. Which of the following publications contains the regulations for using x rays up to 50 MeV?

A. NCRP Report #99
B. NCRP Report #100
C. NCRP Report #102
D. NCRP Report #105

C

245. Which of the following government agencies is responsible for governing the use of radiation?

A. Health, Education and Welfare
B. Food and Drug Administration
C. Nuclear Regulatory Commission
D. Environmental Protection Agency

B

246. The source-to-skin distance in mobile fluoroscopy must NOT be less than how many inches?

A. 6
B. 12
C. 24
D. 36

B

247. What is the dose equivalent limits a pregnant radiologic technologist may receive during the gestation period?

A. 5 mSv (0.5 rem)
B. 10 mSv (1.0 rem)
C. 50 mSv (5.0 rem)
D. 100 mSv (10 rem)

A

248. What is the dose equivalent limits a radiation worker may receive to his/her whole body in one year?

A. 10 mSv (1.0 rem)
B. 50 mSv (5.0 rem)
C. 100 mSv (10 rem)
D. 250 mSv (25 rem)

B

249. A "Radiation Area" warning sign must be visible in areas where the exposure rate exceeds which of these?

A. .05 mSv/hr (5 mrem/hr)
B. .10 mSv/hr (10 mrem/hr)
C. .15 mSv/hr (15 mrem/hr)
D. .20 mSv/hr (20 mrem/hr)

A

250. Which of the following is a responsibility of the Nuclear Regulatory Commission?

1. Set x-ray manufacturing standards
2. Police manufacturing standards
3. Police the field of nuclear medicine

A. 1 only
B. 1 & 2 only
C. 2 & 3 only
D. 1, 2 & 3

D

251. Who is the person in the hospital that is responsible for governing the use of radiation sources?

A. Administrator
B. Radiologist
C. Chief technologist
D. Radiation safety officer

D

252. Who is responsible for routine radiation safety checks in the radiology department?

A. Radiologist
B. Chief technologist
C. Radiographer
D. Qualified expert (e.g., radiation physicist)

D

253. Which of the following topics is covered in NCRP Report #102?

1. Equipment design and use
2. Personnel monitoring
3. Radiation survey procedures

A. 2 only
B. 3 only
C. 1 & 2 only
D. 1, 2 & 3

D

254. Which of the following areas are covered by standards and regulations of x rays?

1. Manufacture and repair of equipment
2. Facility design
3. Personnel qualifications

A. 1 only
B. 2 only
C. 3 only
D. 1, 2 & 3

D

255. Mobile fluoroscopic equipment must have which of the following?

A. VCR capabilities
B. Image intensification
C. T.V. monitoring
D. Solid state circuitry

B

256. The source-to-skin distance for mobile radiography cannot be less than which of the following?

A. 12"
B. 24"
C. 30"
D. 48"

A

257. When operating portable radiographic equipment, the radiographer must be able to stand how far from the patient?

A. 2 feet
B. 3 feet
C. 6 feet
D. 9 feet

C

258. There are two national bodies that set standards for radiography. Which of these is one of them?

A. National Council on Radiation Protection & Measurements
B. Department of Commerce
C. National Bureau of Standards
D. Food and Drug Administration

A

259. A recommendation that is necessary to meet the accepted standards is indicated by the use of which term?

A. Can
B. May
C. Shall
D. Should

C

260. A recommendation that is to be applied when practical is indicated by the use of which of these terms?

A. Can
B. May
C. Shall
D. Should

D

CHAPTER TWO

EQUIPMENT OPERATION

- Fundamentals of Physics (30 questions)
- Electricity (38 questions)
- Magnetic Properties (42 questions)
- Circuits (30 questions)
- X-ray Tube (46 questions)
- X-rays and Their Interactions (36 questions)
- The Atom (20 questions)
- Fluoroscopy (30 questions)
- Digital Imaging (80 questions)

FUNDAMENTALS OF PHYSICS

261. What is the branch of science that deals with matter, energy and their relationship to each other?

A. Radiologic physics
B. Biology
C. Chemistry
D. Physics

D

262. The branch of physics pertaining to the origin and nature of x rays is defined by which of the following?

A. Electronics
B. Quantum mechanics
C. Radiologic physics
D. Physical science

C

263. A body at rest or in uniform motion remains in the same state unless a force is applied describes what?

A. A = F/m
B. For every action there is a reaction
C. Newton's first law of motion
D. Coulomb's law

C

264. What must be applied in order to set a resting body in motion?

1. Potential energy
2. Work
3. Force

A. 1 only
B. 3 only
C. 2 & 3 only
D. 1, 2 & 3

B

265. Which of the following formulas states Newton's second law of motion?

A. F = ma
B. W = Fd
C. $E = mc^2$
D. $K.E. = 1/2mv^2$

A

266. What is the unit of length in the metric MKS system?

A. Meter
B. Liter
C. Kilogram
D. Yard

A

267. What is the unit of mass in the metric MKS system?

A. Ounce
B. Weight
C. Pound
D. Kilogram

D

268. What are the fundamental metric units of physics?

A. Yards, feet and meters
B. Pounds, grams and kilograms
C. Newtons, joules and watts
D. Meters, kilograms and seconds

D

269. What is the formula for converting degrees Fahrenheit to degrees Centigrade?

A. 5/9 (F-32)
B. 9/5 (C+32)
C. 9/5 (F-32)
D. 5/9 (C+32)

A

270. Convert 68 degrees Fahrenheit to degrees Centigrade.

A. 20 degrees
B. 30 degrees
C. 40 degrees
D. 50 degrees

A

271. How many pounds are in a kilogram?

A. 1.1
B. 2.2
C. 3.3
D. 4.4

B

272. How many centimeters are in an inch?

A. 1.63
B. 2.10
C. 2.54
D. 3.46

C

273. Which of the following is incorrect?

A. 1 meter = 100 centimeters
B. 1 centimeter = .01 meters
C. 1 inch = 2.54 centimeters
D. 1 centimeter = 100 millimeters

D

274. Which of the following equals 1 millimeter?

A. 2.54 centimeters
B. .001 meters
C. 10 centimeters
D. 25.4 inches

B

275. How many angstroms are in a meter?

A. 1,000
B. 10,000
C. 1,000,000
D. 10,000,000,000

D

276. What is the push or pull on an object called?

A. Work
B. Force
C. Acceleration
D. Motion

B

277. What is the unit of force?

A. Joule
B. Watt
C. Newton
D. Volt

C

278. Which of the following is the product of force times distance?

A. Work
B. Watt
C. Acceleration
D. Ampere

A

279. What is the definition of energy?

A. Moving or stationary objects
B. Mass times acceleration
C. The rate at which work is done
D. The ability to do work

D

280. The ability of a moving body to do work is called what?

A. Static energy
B. Potential energy
C. Kinetic energy
D. Wave energy

C

281. Which of the following represents a form of stored or potential energy?

A. A flying arrow
B. A falling rock
C. A stretched rubber band
D. A bicycle

C

282. What is the prefix for one million?

A. Kilo
B. Mega
C. Milli
D. Micro

B

283. One thousandth of an ampere would be referred to as what?

A. Centiampere
B. Milliampere
C. Kiloampere
D. Nanoampere

B

284. What is the definition of power?

A. The rate at which work is done
B. The stored energy of an object
C. A body at rest
D. The force of a moving object

A

285. What law states that energy can neither be created nor destroyed, but it can be changed from one form to another?

A. Second Law of Thermodynamics
B. Einstein's Law
C. Joule's Law
D. Law of Conservation of Energy

D

286. What is the unit of power?

A. Watt
B. Joule
C. Ampere
D. Volt

A

287. What does the prefix kilo stand for?

A. 10
B. 100
C. 1,000
D. 1,000,000

C

288. How many centimeters are in a meter?

A. 10
B. 100
C. 1,000
D. 1,000,000

B

289. Which of the following numbers is the same as 10 to the 6th power?

A. 10
B. 100
C. 1,000
D. 1,000,000

D

290. Which of the following numbers is the same as 10 to the -3rd power?

A. 1/10
B. 1/100
C. 1/1,000
D. 1/1,000,000

C

ELECTRICITY

291. What are the two kinds of electrical charges?

A. Ground and ampere
B. Volt and ampere
C. Positive and negative
D. Coulomb and volt

C

292. What is the unit of electrical charge?

A. Ampere
B. Volt
C. Coulomb
D. Farad

C

293. Which of the following statements is true?

A. Unlike charges repel each other
B. Unlike charges attract each other
C. Neutral charges repel each other
D. Like charges attract each other

B

294. When the distance between two charged bodies is cut in half, how much will the force between them increase?

A. 2X
B. 4X
C. 6X
D. 8X

B

295. The work done on a charged particle is measured in which of the following units?

A. Volt
B. Ampere
C. Coulomb
D. Watt

A

296. What determines the quantity of electrons that can be stored in a capacitor?

1. The area of the plates
2. The distance between the plates
3. The material between the plates

A. 1 only
B. 3 only
C. 2 & 3 only
D. 1, 2 & 3

D

297. An electrical charge can be neutralized if it is conducted to what?

A. Ground
B. A metal pipe
C. A magnet
D. A battery

A

298. When an electron is accelerated through a potential difference of 1 volt, how much work is done?

A. 1 Ampere
B. 1 Coulomb
C. 1 Joule
D. 1 Electron volt

D

299. What is a device called that stores electrical charges?

A. Capacitor
B. Ammeter
C. Voltmeter
D. Ground

A

300. What is the unit of capacitance?

A. Volt
B. Ampere
C. Farad
D. Coulomb

C

301. Which of the following is equal to one volt?

A. 1 Joule/Coulomb
B. 1 Ampere/Ohm
C. 1 Ohm/Ampere
D. 1 Ohm/Joule

A

302. Which of the following is NOT related to the force applied to an electrical charge?

A. Voltage
B. Potential difference
C. Electromotive force
D. Amperage

D

303. An excessive amount of electrons at one end of a conductor and a deficiency at the other is known as what?

A. Resistance
B. Amperage
C. Voltage
D. Impedance

C

304. A material that freely allows the flow of electrons is known as what?

A. Conductor
B. Insulator
C. Capacitor
D. Semi-conductor

A

305. The flow of electrons is known as what?

A. Voltage
B. Space charge
C. Current
D. Capacitance

C

306. What is the unit of electrical current?

A. Watt
B. Farad
C. Volt
D. Ampere

D

307. Which of the following causes electrons to move in a conductor?

A. Voltage
B. Amperage
C. Wattage
D. Charge

A

308. Which type of current is supplied by a battery?

A. Direct
B. Pulsating direct
C. Alternating
D. Spiked

A

309. What is the device called that measures electrical current?

A. Capacitor
B. Ammeter
C. Voltmeter
D. Ground

B

310. Which of the following will create the most electrical resistance?

A. A long wire with a small diameter
B. A short wire with a small diameter
C. A long wire with a large diameter
D. A short wire with a large diameter

A

311. Of the following, which will create the least electrical resistance?

A. Copper
B. Aluminum
C. Tungsten
D. Lead

A

312. Which of the following does NOT affect electrical resistance?

A. The length of the conductor
B. The diameter of the conductor
C. The material of the conductor
D. The brand of the conductor

D

313. A material that disallows the flow of electrons is known as what?

A. Conductor
B. Insulator
C. Capacitor
D. Battery

B

314. What law states that the resistance in a circuit is equal to the voltage divided by the current?

A. Coulomb's Law
B. Law of Electrostatics
C. Ohm's Law
D. Newton's Law

C

315. What is the unit for resistance?

A. Volt
B. Watt
C. Ampere
D. Ohm

D

316. According to Ohm's law, what would the voltage be if the resistance is 2 ohm and the current is 4 ampere?

A. 2 volt
B. 4 volt
C. 8 volt
D. 10 volt

C

317. According to Ohm's law, what would the resistance be if the voltage is 110 volt and the current is 5 ampere?

A. 22 ohm
B. 55 ohm
C. 220 ohm
D. 550 ohm

A

318. According to Ohm's law, what would the current be if the voltage is 12 volt and the resistance is 1.5 ohm?

A. 2 ampere
B. 4 ampere
C. 6 ampere
D. 8 ampere

D

319. Which of the following statements concerning a series circuit is true?

1. Amperage remains constant throughout
2. Voltage remains constant throughout
3. Resistance is always constant

A. 1 only
B. 2 only
C. 1 & 3 only
D. 1, 2 & 3

A

320. 2 ohm, 4 ohm and 6 ohm resistors connected in series would result in a total resistance of how many ohms?

A. 4
B. 8
C. 12
D. 16

C

321. How are parallel resistors connected?

A. Side-by-side
B. End-to-end
C. Side-to-end
D. In a coil

A

322. Parallel resistors of 3 ohm and 6 ohm would result in a total resistance of how many ohm?

A. 1
B. 2
C. 3
D. 4

B

323. What electrical device will prevent equipment damage if currents get too high?

A. Circuit breaker
B. Capacitor
C. Voltmeter
D. Ground

A

324. A device whose electrical resistance may be varied is called what?

A. Breaker switch
B. Rheostat
C. Transformer
D. Rectifier

B

325. What is the unit of electrical power?

A. Ohm
B. Farad
C. Watt
D. Joule

C

326. What is the formula for electrical power?

A. P = VR
B. P = IR
C. P = W/T
D. P = VI

D

327. Which of the following moves in a conductor?

A. Positive charges
B. Negative charges
C. Neutral particles
D. Atomic nuclei

B

328. A technique of 70 kVp at 400 mA produces how many watts of power?

A. 280 watts
B. 2800 watts
C. 28,000 watts
D. 280,000 watts

C

MAGNETIC PROPERTIES

329. What is a material called that will attract small pieces of iron?

A. Solenoid
B. Helix
C. Magnet
D. Compound

C

330. Every magnet has two poles. What are they called?

A. East and west
B. East and north
C. North and west
D. North and south

D

331. What are the magnetic lines called that surround a magnet?

A. Flux lines
B. Swirls
C. Topographic
D. Latitude

A

332. Which of the following determines the strength of a magnetic field?

A. The magnet's diameter
B. The number of flux lines in an area
C. The spin of the magnet
D. How tightly the magnet is wrapped

B

333. How would cutting the distance between two magnets in half effect the attraction force between them?

A. It would double
B. It would increase four times
C. It would be halved
D. It would not change

B

334. In which direction do magnetic flux lines travel?

A. North pole to south pole
B. South pole to north pole
C. East pole to west pole
D. There is no specific direction

A

335. What surrounds every electrical current?

A. Insulation
B. Sound waves
C. Magnetic field
D. Electromagnetic radiation

C

336. Which of the following happens when the current in a conductor increases?

A. Magnetic field strength increases
B. Magnetic field strength decreases
C. Resistance increases
D. Magnetic field changes direction

A

337. Which of the following rules will determine the direction of the magnetic field around an electrical current?

A. Left hand rule
B. Right hand rule
C. Left hand thumb rule
D. Right hand thumb rule

C

338. According to the left hand thumb rule, which direction would the magnetic field be if the current is toward you?

A. Clockwise
B. Counterclockwise
C. Vertical
D. Horizontal

A

339. What is a spring shaped coil of wire called?

A. Solenoid
B. Tap turn
C. Transformer
D. Helix

D

340. What is a current carrying coil of wire called?

A. Solenoid
B. Rectifier
C. Spring
D. Rheostat

A

341. What is it called when a solenoid has an iron core in its center?

A. Electroflux
B. Electrolux
C. Electromagnet
D. Diamagnet

C

342. What are materials called that are strongly attracted to a magnet?

A. Diamagnetic
B. Paramagnetic
C. Ferromagnetic
D. Steromagnetic

C

343. What are materials called that are NOT attracted to a magnet?

A. Paramagnetic
B. Non-magnetic
C. Diamagnetic
D. Sumagnetic

B

344. What are materials called that are weakly attracted to a magnet?

A. Sumagnetic
B. Diamagnetic
C. Paramagnetic
D. Ferromagnetic

C

345. How are the north poles of two magnets going to affect each other?

A. They will attract
B. They will repel
C. They will change polarization
D. They will not be affected

B

346. Materials that are easily magnetized and demagnetized are said to have a high ____.

A. Retentivity
B. Repelability
C. Permeability
D. Attractability

C

347. How will the north pole and the south pole of two magnets affect each other?

A. They will attract
B. They will repel
C. They will change polarization
D. They will not be affected

A

348. Which of the following happens when a wire moves through a magnetic field?

1. An electromotive force is induced
2. The resistance in the wire increases
3. The magnetic field disappears

A. 1 only
B. 2 only
C. 2 & 3 only
D. 1, 2 & 3

A

349. Maximum induction will occur when a conductor cuts a magnetic field at what angle?

A. 0 degrees
B. 45 degrees
C. 90 degrees
D. 180 degrees

C

350. Materials that are difficult to magnetize and demagnetize are said to have a high _____.

A. Retentivity
B. Repelability
C. Permeability
D. Attractability

A

351. A coil of wire rotating through a magnetic field produces an electric current. What does this describe?

A. Motor
B. Rectifier
C. Generator
D. Transformer

C

352. How can voltage be induced into a conductor?

1. Move a wire through a magnetic field
2. Move a magnetic field across a wire
3. Place a wire in a varying magnetic field

A. 1 only
B. 3 only
C. 1 & 3 only
D. 1, 2 & 3

D

353. A _____ works by sending an alternating current through a coil of wire that has been placed within a magnetic field.

A. Motor
B. Transformer
C. Generator
D. Solenoid

A

354. What is it called when a current is induced in a secondary coil by simply changing the current in the primary coil?

A. Back EMF
B. Mutual induction
C. Resistance
D. Magnetism

B

355. What type of transformer has more turns of wire in the secondary side than in the primary side?

A. Step-up
B. Step-down
C. Delta
D. Deltoid

A

356. What type of transformer core is most widely used in radiographic equipment?

A. Air core
B. Open core
C. Closed core
D. Shell type

D

357. What determines the transformer ratio?

A. Size of wire
B. Turns of wire
C. Type of wire
D. Current in wire

B

358. Which type of transformer core is most efficient?

A. Air core
B. Open core
C. Closed core
D. Shell type

D

359. If the voltage is stepped-up, what happens to the current in the secondary side of the transformer?

A. Increases
B. Decreases
C. Stays the same
D. Stepped-up

B

360. As magnetic domains rearrange in a transformer, heat is produced. What is this energy loss called?

A. Copper losses
B. Eddy currents
C. Hysteresis losses
D. Energy swells

C

361. Which of the following materials would make the best transformer core?

A. Plastic
B. Aluminum
C. Wood
D. Soft iron

D

362. What are the swirling currents called that are induced in transformers and produce heat losses?

A. Eddy currents
B. Transformer currents
C. Lamination currents
D. Hysteresis currents

A

363. The number of cycles per second that are associated with an alternating current are known as the current's what?

A. Frequency
B. Period
C. Wavelength
D. Amplitude

A

364. In a 60 cycle alternating current, how many alternations are there every second?

A. 30
B. 60
C. 90
D. 120

D

365. How are alternating current values usually expressed?

A. Peak values
B. Average values
C. Mean values
D. RMS values

D

366. What is the major reason for using alternating current?

A. X-ray tubes require it
B. Rectifiers cannot work without it
C. Transformers cannot operate without it
D. Current cannot flow without it

C

367. An electric current that continually changes directions is known as what type of current?

A. Direct
B. Alternating
C. Reversible
D. Stationary

B

368. If a step-up transformer has a turns ratio of 1:1000, what will the output voltage be if the input voltage is 50 V?

A. 50 V
B. 50 kV
C. 500 V
D. 500 kV

B

369. If a step-down transformer has a turns ratio of 1:10, what will the output voltage be if the input voltage is 220 V?

A. 22 V
B. 22 kV
C. 220 V
D. 220 kV

A

370. If the peak kilovoltage on a single phase unit is set on 100 kVp, what will the R.M.S. value be?

A. 50.5 kV
B. 70.7 kV
C. 100 kV
D. 141 kV

B

CIRCUITS

371. The changing of alternating current to direct current is known as what?

A. Transformation
B. Rectification
C. Conversion
D. Electrification

B

372. What is the name of the closed path over which electric current flows?

A. Circuit
B. Differential
C. Airway
D. Ampere

A

373. What is a device called that allows current to flow in only one direction?

A. Insulator
B. Conductor
C. Semiconductor
D. Capacitor

C

374. Which type of rectification will supply the x-ray tube with the greatest power?

A. Self
B. Half-wave
C. Full-wave
D. Sine-wave

C

375. What is the voltage supplied to the autotransformer called?

A. Peak voltage
B. Effective voltage
C. Average voltage
D. Line voltage

D

376. What controls the incoming voltage to the autotransformer?

A. Rectifier
B. Main breaker switch
C. Fuses
D. Timer

B

377. Which of the following is the most accurate timer?

A. Impulse timer
B. Synchronous timer
C. Sine-wave timer
D. Electronic timer

D

378. Tapping windings of the autotransformer to supply voltage to the step-up transformer is the purpose of which of these?

A. kVp selector
B. Voltmeter
C. Voltage compensator
D. Rheostat

A

379. If line voltage changes because of demands by other users, adjustments must be made in which of the following?

A. Step-up transformer
B. Rheostat
C. Voltage compensator
D. Prereading voltmeter

C

380. Which of the following is placed in the circuit in case of current changes during the exposure?

A. Transformer
B. Breaker switch
C. Choke coil
D. Rectifier

B

381. Where in the x-ray circuit is the timer located?

A. In the secondary circuit
B. Between the autotransformer and the step-up transformer
C. Before the step-down transformer
D. Between the rectifier and the x-ray tube

B

382. Which of the following is an advantage of three-phase equipment over single-phase equipment?

A. Less expensive
B. Can achieve shorter exposure times
C. Easier to operate
D. Produces less exposure

B

383. The spinning top test can be used to determine the accuracy of which of the following?

A. Rectification circuit
B. Autotransformer
C. Cooling circuit
D. Low voltage circuit

A

384. What device would be used when the milliamperage is set on the control panel?

A. Milliammeter
B. Rheostat
C. Autotransformer
D. Step-up transformer

B

385. Which of the following meters does NOT register until an x-ray exposure is made?

A. Prereading kilovoltmeter
B. Prereading ammeter
C. Kilovoltmeter
D. Milliammeter

D

386. A 1/10th second exposure is made on a full-wave rectified, single- phase generator. A spinning top will show how many dots?

A. 6
B. 8
C. 10
D. 12

D

387. Which of the following types of current supplies the x-ray tube?

A. Alternating current
B. Direct current
C. Pulsating direct current
D. Saturated current

C

388. What effect does adjusting the filament control have on the production of x rays?

A. Controls the quantity
B. Controls the energy
C. Controls the quality
D. Controls the penetrating power

A

389. Which of the following is the current indicated by the milliammeter?

A. Saturation current
B. Tube current
C. Rectified current
D. Maximum current

B

390. The incoming line voltage is 220 volts. 55% of the turns on the autotransformer are used. What is the voltage sent to the step-up transformer?

A. 121 volts
B. 121 kilovolts
C. 220 volts
D. 220 kilovolts

A

391. How many solid state rectifiers are needed to produce a single-phase, full-wave rectified current?

A. 1
B. 2
C. 3
D. 4

D

392. If a full-wave rectified current has 60 cycles per second, how many pulses per second cross the x-ray tube?

A. 60
B. 90
C. 120
D. 180

C

393. A solid-state rectifier is primarily made of which of the following substances?

A. Aluminum
B. Arsenic
C. Silicon
D. Iron

C

394. To produce equal density and contrast, exposure to the patient with three-phase equipment is _____ compared to single-phase.

A. Equal
B. Greater
C. Less
D. Double

A

395. DEXA is the abbreviation for _____.

A. Dual Energy X-ray Attenuation
B. Density Effects of X-ray Absorption
C. Direct Evaluation of Xanthoma Abnormality
D. Dual Energy X-ray Absorptiometry

D

396. Which of the following is NOT an advantage of automatic exposure control (AEC)?

1. Eliminates the need to select mAs
2. Duplicates radiographic densities
3. More latitude in patient positioning

A. 1 only
B. 3 only
C. 2 & 3 only
D. 1, 2 & 3

B

397. Why are three-phase generators more efficient at producing x rays than single-phase generators?

A. Shorter times are possible
B. Voltage never drops to zero
C. Current travels faster
D. Less heat units are produced

B

398. Which of the following is NOT essential to the operation of automatic exposure controls (AEC)?

A. Capacitor
B. Electron emitting device
C. Back-up timer
D. Image intensifier

D

399. In the x-ray circuit diagram below, the letter "A" is directly above which of the following circuit components?

A. Autotransformer
B. Step-down or filament transformer
C. Kilovoltage indicator
D. Milliamperage selector

B

400. In the x-ray circuit diagram below, the letter "B" is directly above which of the following circuit components?

A. Timer
B. Step-up transformer
C. Milliammeter
D. Rectification circuit

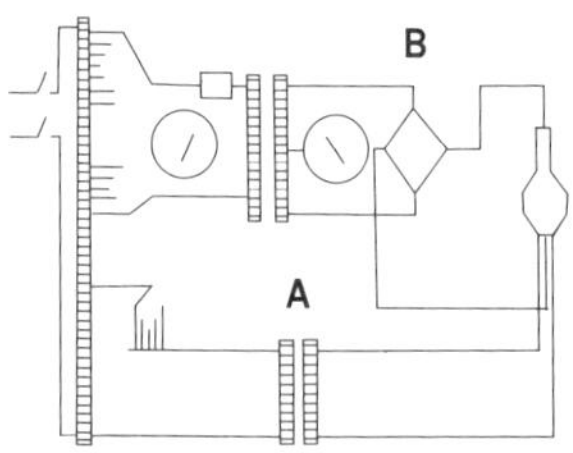

D

X-RAY TUBE

401. The target of an x-ray tube is made from what metal?

A. Lead
B. Copper
C. Tungsten
D. Molybdenum

C

402. Why is an x-ray tube immersed in oil?

A. Reduce noise
B. Prevent sparking
C. Insulation
D. Filtration

C

403. What causes most x-ray tube failures?

A. Heating of the anode
B. Multiple exposures
C. Cracked glass
D. Excessive heat

D

404. What type of primary radiation is produced when the x-ray tube voltage is below 70 kVp?

A. Characteristic
B. Bremsstrahlung
C. Compton
D. Scatter

B

405. What type of motor drives the rotating anode?

A. Synchronous
B. Induction
C. Direct current
D. Inductive reactance

B

406. Which part of the x-ray tube has the filament wires and focusing cup?

A. Cathode
B. Anode
C. Housing
D. Impregnated glass

A

407. As kilovoltage is applied, the electrons are accelerated toward which part of the x-ray tube?

A. Cathode
B. Anode
C. Window
D. Stem

B

408. Which of the following will produce the least load on an x-ray tube?

A. High kVp, high mAs
B. High kVp, low mAs
C. Low kVp, high mAs
D. All will produce an equal load

B

409. Which of the following is required of a target metal in an x-ray tube?

1. Ability to conduct heat
2. High atomic number
3. High melting point

A. 2 only
B. 1 & 3 only
C. 2 & 3 only
D. 1, 2 & 3

D

410. Which of the following increases the penetrating power of the x-ray beam?

A. Milliamperage
B. Seconds
C. Kilovoltage
D. Distance

C

411. What is the area of the x-ray target called that is struck by electrons?

A. Actual focal spot
B. Effective focal spot
C. Rotating focal spot
D. Heating track

A

412. When electrons strike the target of an x-ray tube, most of their energy is converted to what?

A. Heat
B. Light
C. X rays
D. Gamma rays

A

413. Which of the following is the negative terminal of the x-ray tube?

A. Cathode
B. Anode
C. Target
D. Tungsten disk

A

414. What are x-ray tubes called that have two filament wires?

A. Dual focus tubes
B. Double cathode tubes
C. Triode tubes
D. Field emission tubes

A

415. How many kilovolts is equal to 75,000 volts?

A. 7.5 kV
B. 75 kV
C. 750 kV
D. 75,000 kV

B

416. The formula, mA x kVp x time, is used to determine which of the following?

A. Safe exposures
B. Penetrating power
C. Heat units
D. Exposure in Roentgens

C

417. The small craters in the target of the anode of an x-ray tube are known as what?

A. Hot spots
B. Pitting
C. Melting points
D. Blistering

B

418. What is used to focus the electron stream toward the target of the anode?

A. Lead collar
B. Focusing cup
C. Copper anode
D. Focusing lens

B

419. Electrons travel in an x-ray tube from _____ to _____.

A. Target, anode
B. Target, window
C. Cathode, anode
D. Anode, cathode

C

420. Which of the following is the filtration that is manufactured into the x-ray tube?

A. Added filtration
B. Compensating filtration
C. Inherent filtration
D. Adjusted filtration

C

421. What determines the quantity of electrons that will be accelerated across the x-ray tube?

A. Focal spot size
B. Kilovoltage
C. Anode speed
D. Heating of the filament

D

422. During thermionic emission a cloud of electrons surround the filament. What is this electron cloud called?

A. Space charge
B. Electron charge
C. Charged cloud
D. Filament charge

A

423. If used properly, will an x-ray tube last forever?

A. Yes
B. No, the anode will disintegrate
C. No, the filament wire will break
D. No, the focus will melt away

C

424. How fast do high speed anodes rotate?

A. 1,500 RPM
B. 3,400 RPM
C. 5,000 RPM
D. 10,000 RPM

D

425. Which of the following causes pitting of the x-ray tube target?

A. Using both filaments at once
B. Using the small focus all the time
C. Moderate overloading of the tube
D. Malfunction of high speed rotor

C

426. According to the line focus principle, the effective focal spot is ____ than the actual focal spot.

A. Smaller
B. Larger
C. Brighter
D. Sharper

A

427. As the x-ray tube gets older, what happens to the temperature of the filament?

A. Increases
B. Decreases
C. Varies
D. Remains the same

A

428. Which of the following would NOT be found in an x-ray tube?

A. Focusing cup
B. Filament wire
C. Rotor
D. Rotor button

D

429. As electrons are accelerated across the x-ray tube they are referred to as which of the following?

A. Filament current
B. Cathode current
C. Anode current
D. Tube current

D

430. What is the purpose of the anode in an x-ray tube?

A. Emits electrons
B. Decelerates electrons
C. Focuses electrons
D. Repels electrons

B

431. What is the purpose of a window in an x-ray tube?

A. For watching the x ray production
B. For the emission of x rays
C. To stop all harmful x rays
D. Allows light to pass for centering

B

432. What effect will increasing the kVp have on the production of x rays?

A. Their number will increase
B. Their speed will increase
C. Their energy will increase
D. Their wavelength will increase

C

433. When will a space charge be present in the x-ray tube?

A. Never, its outside of the tube
B. Whenever the rotor is engaged
C. Whenever the machine is turned on
D. There is always a space charge

B

434. Which of the following is NOT needed to produce x rays?

A. Availability of electrons
B. Electrons set in high speed motion
C. Electrons stopped suddenly
D. Focusing cup

D

435. What is the formula for heat units in a three-phase, six-pulse, x-ray unit?

A. mA x kVp x time
B. mA x kVp x time x 1.35
C. mA x kVp x time x 2
D. mA x kVp x time x 3.33

B

436. Why is an x-ray tube made of Pyrex glass?

A. To prevent breakage if dropped
B. To better withstand heat
C. A lead tube would be too heavy
D. For a clearer passage of the x rays

B

437. When electrons strike the anode of an x-ray tube, how much of their energy is converted to x rays?

A. Less than 1%
B. 10%
C. 50%
D. More than 99%

A

438. Which of the following parts would make up the cathode end of the x-ray tube?

A. Filaments and rotor
B. Rotor and rotating disk
C. Filaments and focusing cup
D. Rotor, rotating disk and target

C

439. In a modern, rotating anode x-ray tube, which of the following will coat the tungsten disk?

A. Tungsten rhenium alloy
B. Tungsten molybdenum alloy
C. Tungsten copper alloy
D. Tungsten lead alloy

A

440. During an exposure, what electrical charge is placed on the anode?

A. Negative
B. Positive
C. Covalent
D. Neutral

B

441. What is the process of "boiling off" electrons called?

A. Space charge production
B. Electron emission
C. Thermionic emission
D. Heat production

C

442. From what metal are the filament wires in radiographic tubes made?

A. Molybdenum
B. Lead
C. Copper
D. Tungsten

D

443. Which of the following is NOT related to the others?

A. Rotor
B. Target
C. Filament
D. Tungsten disk

C

444. In what units is filament current measured?

A. Voltage
B. Kilovoltage
C. Amperage
D. Milliamperage

C

445 Which of the following is smallest?

A. Space charge
B. Actual focal spot
C. Effective focal spot
D. Target

C

446. Why is the x-ray tube made from lead impregnated glass and encased in a lead housing?

A. Prevent electrical shock
B. Prevent leakage radiation
C. Allow for thermal conduction
D. Protection from breakage

B

X RAYS AND THEIR INTERACTIONS

447. Which of the following is NOT a property of x rays?

A. Travel at the speed of light
B. Travel in straight lines
C. Produce biological changes
D. Negatively charged

D

448. Which of the following electromagnetic waves has the shortest wavelength?

A. Visible light
B. Radar
C. X ray
D. Ultraviolet

C

449. Which of the following is a byproduct of photoelectric absorption?

1. Bremsstrahlung radiation
2. Photoelectron
3. Recoil electron

A. 1 only
B. 2 only
C. 2 & 3 only
D. 1, 2 & 3

B

450. Which of the following does NOT affect the attenuation of an x-ray beam?

A. Scatter
B. Absorption
C. Distance
D. Speed

D

451. When were x rays discovered?

A. November 8, 1895
B. November 5, 1898
C. January 13, 1896
D. January 6, 1913

A

452. What is it called when a primary photon changes direction but NOT energy?

A. Coherent (classical) scatter
B. Modified scattering
C. Compton effect
D. Photoelectric absorption

A

453. Which of the following interactions does NOT occur under 125 kVp?

A. Compton effect
B. Pair production
C. Photoelectric absorption
D. Coherent (classical) scatter

B

454. Which of the following would best describe the wavelengths of a diagnostic x-ray beam?

A. Homogeneous
B. Heterogeneous
C. Monochromatic
D. Monoenergetic

B

455. Which of the following will NOT reduce the intensity of an x-ray beam?

A. Compton effect
B. Photoelectric absorption
C. Characteristic effect
D. Pair production

C

456. Which of the following would describe an x-ray photon?

A. High speed electron
B. High speed neutron
C. High speed proton
D. High speed bundle of energy

D

457. Which of the following is responsible for most of the scatter radiation in the diagnostic range?

A. Photoelectric absorption
B. Bremsstrahlung radiation
C. Compton effect
D. Photon skipping

C

458. What characterizes the Compton effect?

A. Recoil electron
B. Total absorption of primary photon
C. Photoelectron
D. Primary photon does not lose energy

A

459. X rays are classified as what type of radiation?

A. Expansion
B. Sound
C. Destructive
D. Electromagnetic

D

460. The quality of an x-ray beam refers to what?

A. Number of x rays
B. Exposure rate
C. Energy of x rays
D. Ability to ionize

C

461. X rays are very much the same as which of the following?

A. Alpha particles
B. Beta particles
C. Gamma rays
D. Sting rays

C

462. As the wavelength of an x ray increases, what happens to its frequency?

A. Increases
B. Decreases
C. Changes directions
D. Remains the same

B

463. Biological changes caused by x rays are the result of which of the following?

A. Ionization
B. Excitation
C. Attenuation
D. Evolution

A

464. Which of the following results in the total absorption of the primary x-ray photon?

A. Compton effect
B. Coherent (classical) scatter
C. Pair production
D. Photoelectric absorption

D

465. The half-value layer is an expression of the _____ of an x-ray beam.

A. Quantity
B. Quality
C. Refraction
D. Ionization

B

466. Which of the following has the greatest effect on radiographic contrast?

A. Compton effect
B. Coherent (classical) scatter
C. Pair production
D. Photoelectric absorption

A

467. What determines the wavelength of an x ray?

A. Milliamperage
B. Time
C. Kilovoltage
D. Distance

C

468. Which of the following describes the x rays that are produced in the radiographic tube?

A. Remnant (exit) radiation
B. Primary radiation
C. Secondary radiation
D. Scatter radiation

B

469. In the normal diagnostic range, which of the following interactions will occur most often?

A. Compton effect
B. Photoelectric absorption
C. Coherent (classical) scatter
D. Pair production

A

470. What is the unit for radiation exposure in air?

A. Erg
B. Joule
C. Roentgen
D. Rad

C

471. In the normal diagnostic range, what is the wavelength range of the x rays?

A. 1 to 5 inches
B. 1 to 5 centimeters
C. .1 to .5 angstroms
D. .1 to .5 millimeters

C

472. Which of the following is the speed of x rays?

A. 186,000 miles/second
B. 186,000 feet/second
C. 186,000 miles/hour
D. 186,000 meters/minute

A

473. Which of the following is equal in all electromagnetic radiations?

A. Wavelength
B. Frequency
C. Amplitude
D. Speed

D

474. The maximum x-ray energy will be equal to which of the following?

A. mA
B. mAs
C. kVp
D. Time

C

475. How many angstroms are in a meter?

A. 1,000,00
B. 100,000,000
C. 10,000,000,000
D. 1,000,000,000,000

C

476. Which of the following represents a high energy, x-ray photon?

A. Short wavelength
B. Long wavelength
C. Low frequency
D. High speed

A

477. Which of the following describes the radiation that makes up the x ray beam after it has traversed the patient?

A. Remnant (exit) radiation
B. Primary radiation
C. Secondary radiation
D. Scatter radiation

A

478. What is it called when the x-ray beam is reduced in intensity as it traverses an object?

A. Ionization
B. Attenuation
C. Quantization
D. Elimination

B

479. During the Compton effect, x rays most often interact with which of the following?

A. Outer shell electrons
B. Inner shell electrons
C. The nucleus
D. Protons

A

480. Which of the following types of primary radiation cannot be produced at tube potentials less than 70 keV?

A. Bremsstrahlung
B. Characteristic
C. Primary
D. Secondary

B

481. What is the distance between two wave crests of an electromagnetic wave called?

A. Wave velocity
B. Wave amplitude
C. Wavelength
D. Frequency

C

482. Which type of radiation is produced when a high speed electron is slowed down or suddenly stopped?

A. Bremsstrahlung
B. Characteristic
C. Remnant (exit)
D. Scatter

A

THE ATOM

483. What is the process called that changes a neutral atom into an electrically charged atom?

A. Fission
B. Fusion
C. Electrification
D. Ionization

D

484. Which of the following refers to the number of electrons in the outer shell of an electron?

A. Valence number
B. Atomic number
C. Atomic weight
D. Electrical charge

A

485. What are the particles called that continuously circle the nucleus of an atom?

A. Neutrons
B. Electrons
C. Positrons
D. Protons

B

486. Which of the following is correct concerning a neutral atom?

A. Same number of protons as electrons
B. Same number of protons as neutrons
C. Same number of neutrons as electrons
D. No subatomic particles

A

487. Which of the following describes a proton?

A. No mass and no charge
B. No mass and positive charge
C. Mass and no charge
D. Mass and positive charge

D

488. The mass number of an atom is equal to which of the following?

A. The number of protons
B. The number of neutrons
C. The number of protons and neutrons
D. The number of protons and electrons

C

489. Which of the following subatomic particles is the largest?

A. Proton
B. Electron
C. Neutron
D. Neutrino

C

490. Which particle in the nucleus of an atom has no charge?

A. Neutron
B. Proton
C. Electron
D. Ion

A

491. The atomic number of an atom is equal to which of the following?

A. Number of protons
B. Number of neutrons
C. Number of protons and neutrons
D. Number of protons and electrons

A

492. What does one have when all the elements are arranged in a series according to their atomic numbers?

A. Rating chart
B. Characteristic curve
C. Isotope curve
D. Periodic chart

D

493. What are charged atoms called?

A. Isotopes
B. Ions
C. Isomers
D. Electrons

B

494. Which of the following describes an electron?

A. No mass and no charge
B. No mass and negative charge
C. Mass and no charge
D. Mass and negative charge

D

495. What is the energy called that attracts the electrons to the nucleus of an atom?

A. Natural energy
B. Nuclear energy
C. Binding energy
D. Electron energy

C

496. How many electrons may occupy the M-shell of an atom?

A. 2
B. 8
C. 18
D. 28

C

497. Which of the following would be found in the nucleus of an atom?

1. Proton
2. Electron
3. Neutron

A. 1 only
B. 2 only
C. 1 & 3 only
D. 1, 2 & 3

C

498. If a neutral atom has an atomic number of 10, then how many electrons will it have?

A. 2
B. 6
C. 10
D. 12

C

499. Which of the following pertains to atoms that have their outer electron shell completely filled?

A. Purely electrified
B. Chemically inert
C. Strongly ionized
D. Tightly bonded

B

500. What type of bond holds atoms together by sharing their outer electrons?

A. Covalent
B. Ionic
C. Energetic
D. Characteristic

A

501. If an atom obtains an additional electron, what kind of charge will that ion have?

A. Neutral
B. Positive
C. Negative
D. Attractive

C

502. Who is given credit for describing what an atom looks like?

A. Neils Bohr
B. Albert Einstein
C. Charles Darwin
D. Hans Oersted

A

FLUOROSCOPY

503. What is the purpose of fluoroscopy?

A. To view static anatomy
B. To view dynamic anatomy
C. To view transaxial anatomy
D. To view internal organs

B

504. In a stationary fluoroscopic unit, where is the fluoroscopic x-ray tube located?

A. Under the table
B. Over the table
C. In the fluoroscopic tower
D. The fluoroscopic x-ray tube and the radiographic x-ray tube are the same

A

505. What is the normal tube current during fluoroscopy?

A. 1 to 5 mA
B. 5 to 10 mA
C. 50 to 100 mA
D. 100 to 500 mA

A

506. During fluoroscopy, which of the following is correct?

1. Increasing kVp produces a longer scale of contrast
2. Increasing mA lowers patient dose
3. Increasing spot filming lowers patient dose

A. 1 only
B. 3 only
C. 1 & 2 only
D. 1 & 3 only

A

507. What conversion occurs in the image at the input phosphor of an image intensifier tube?

A. Light is converted to electrons
B. X rays are converted to electrons
C. Electrons are converted to visible light
D. X rays are converted to visible light

D

508. What conversion occurs in the image at the photocathode of an image intensifier tube?

A. Light is converted to electrons
B. X rays are converted to electrons
C. Electrons are converted to visible light
D. X rays are converted to visible light

A

509. What is photoemission?

A. The emission of electrons
B. The emission of electrons from a heated wire
C. The emission of electrons from the photocathode
D. The emission of electrons from the input phosphor

C

510. What conversion occurs in the image at the output phosphor of an image intensifier tube?

A. Light is converted to electrons
B. X rays are converted to electrons
C. Electrons are converted to visible light
D. X rays are converted to visible light

C

511. At what stage of image intensified fluoroscopy is the number of photons lowest?

A. Entering the input phosphor
B. Leaving the input phosphor
C. Entering the output phosphor
D. Leaving the output phosphor

A

512. Which comes first in image intensified fluoroscopy?

A. Photocathode
B. Electrostatic focusing lenses
C. Cesium iodide screen
D. Zinc cadmium sulfide screen

C

513. Which comes last in image intensified fluoroscopy?

A. Photocathode
B. Electrostatic focusing lenses
C. Cesium iodide screen
D. Zinc cadmium sulfide screen

D

514. What are the functions of the electrostatic lenses in an image intensification tube?

1. Focus the electrons from the photocathode
2. Increase the speed of the electrons
3. Condense the image to increase its brightness

A. 1 & 2 only
B. 1 & 3 only
C. 2 & 3 only
D. 1, 2 and 3

D

515. What is the process called when an image intensifier tube makes a dim image brighter?

A. Brightness gain
B. Flux gain
C. Maxification gain
D. Minification gain

A

516. Which of the following will affect the total brightness of an image intensification tube?

1. Flux gain
2. Minification gain
3. Primary beam intensity

A. 1 & 2 only
B. 1 & 3 only
C. 2 & 3 only
D. 1, 2 & 3

D

517. The image intensifier's input phosphor differs from the output phosphor in what way?

A. Is much larger
B. Emits electrons, where the output phosphor emits light
C. Absorbs electrons, where the output phosphor absorbs light
D. Is a fixed size, where the output phosphor's size can vary

A

518. The brightness level of the fluoroscopic image can vary with which of the following?

1. mA
2. Kvp
3. Patient size

A. 1 only
B. 1 & 2 only
C. 2 & 3 only
D. 1, 2 & 3

D

519. Which of the following describes the fluoroscopic system designed to maintain a constant image brightness?

A. Automatic brightness control (ABC)
B. Automatic exposure control (AEC)
C. Automatic collimation
D. Anatomically programmed radiography

A

520. Automatic brightness control (ABC) is designed to compensate for changes in which of the following?

A. Examination time
B. Technique selection
C. Patient positioning
D. Patient dose

C

521. The flux gain of an image intensifier tube increases with an increase in which of the following?

A. mA
B. kVp
C. Input phosphor size
D. Tube voltage

A

522. What happens when a multifocus image intensifier tube is operated in the magnification mode?

A. Patient dose is reduced
B. Recorded detail is reduced
C. A larger area of the patient is seen
D. The electron focal point is closer to the input phosphor

D

523. When using a multifocus image intensifier tube in the magnification mode:

A. resolution is improved.
B. a longer scale of contrast is produced.
C. patient exposure is decreased.
D. the field of view is increased.

A

524. When using a 25/17/12 image intensifier tube, which of the following is true?

A. Resolution is best in the 25 cm mode
B. There are three different input phosphors
C. Resolution is best in the 17 cm mode
D. The field of view is largest in the 25 cm mode

D

525. If the radiologist you worked with requested a TV image with sharp detail, what type of TV camera would you recommend purchasing?

A. Vidicon
B. Plumbicon
C. Zorocon
D. Zoomocon

A

526. How is the electron beam in a television camera tube produced?

A. Thermionic emission
B. Cathode emission
C. Electroemission
D. Photoemission

A

527. The electron beam in a television camera tube is controlled by which of the following?

1. Steering coils
2. Accelerator grids
3. Control grid

A. 1 only
B. 1 & 3 only
C. 2 & 3 only
D. 1, 2 & 3

D

528. The target assembly of a television camera tube consists of which of the following?

1. Window
2. Signal plate
3. Target plate

A. 1 & 2 only
B. 1 & 3 only
C. 2 & 3 only
D. 1, 2 & 3

D

529. Which of the following is photoconductive?

A. Window
B. Signal plate
C. Target plate
D. Electron gun

C

530. Which component of the television monitor transfers the video signal into a visible image?

A. Electron beam
B. Aluminum reflector
C. Anode
D. Fluorescent screen

D

531. Which of the following fluoroscopic image recording systems is capable of recording dynamic images?

A. 70 mm roll film camera
B. 105 mm chip film camera
C. Cassette spot filming
D. VCR

D

532. The advantages of spot film cameras over cassette spot films include which of the following?

1. Decreased patient dose
2. Decreased heat load
3. Shortened exam times

A. 1 only
B. 3 only
C. 2 & 3 only
D. 1, 2 & 3

D

DIGITAL IMAGING

533. When referring to digital imaging, what does the term digital mean?

A. Computer generated images
B. Computer enhanced images
C. Using numbers to compute information
D. Radiographing digits

C

534. A typical digital radiograph contains _____ megabytes of information.

A. .13
B. .52
C. 5.1
D. 7.5

D

535. Which of the following are advantages of digital systems over film-screen systems?

1. Increased dynamic range
2. Higher spatial resolution
3. More contrast resolution

A. 1 only
B. 1 & 3 only
C. 2 & 3 only
D. 1, 2 & 3

B

536. The quality of a digital image depends on which of the following?

1. Histogram
2. Look-up table
3. Display monitor

A. 1 & 2 only
B. 1 & 3 only
C. 2 & 3 only
D. 1, 2 & 3

D

537. What does it mean to direct capture a digital image?

A. The digital image is captured by the printer
B. A CT or MRI image is reconstructed
C. The film digitizer copies the radiograph
D. The x-ray image is captured directly by a detector array

D

538. Which of the following terms is used to describe long-term storage of digital images and documents?

A. Film filing
B. Storage
C. Archive
D. Warehouse

C

539. Computers operate using a binary machine language. This language uses binary digits to compute data. A binary digit is referred to as what?

A. Bit
B. Byte
C. Digit
D. Code

A

540. Which of the following temporarily stores data in the computer?

A. Random Access Memory (RAM)
B. Read Only Memory (ROM)
C. Extended Memory
D. Secondary Memory

A

541. A hospital's plan to periodically backup archived files is known as what?

A. CYA plan
B. Disaster recovery plan
C. PACS protocol
D. Archiving the archives

B

542. Which of the following is a universal standard that allows various digital imaging devices to work together within a network no matter who the manufacturer?

A. TCP/IP
B. DICOM
C. PACS
D. NIC

B

543. The binary code for the decimal number 18 is which of the following?

A. 1001
B. 1010
C. 10001
D. 10010

D

544. The ability to digitally record a small object, its accuracy and its clarity, defines which of the following?

A. Recorded detail
B. Spatial resolution
C. Definition
D. Detail

B

545. What does the acronym R.A.I.D. stand for?

A. Radiology Analysis and Information Data
B. Recall And Input Device
C. Random Access Information Data
D. Redundant Array of Independent Disks

D

546. Each cell of an image matrix is called what?

A. A square
B. A pixel
C. An element
D. A byte

B

547. Spatial resolution in digital imaging is determined by which of the following?

A. Focal spot size
B. Density and contrast
C. Matrix size
D. Matrix size and the size of the field of view

D

548. One of the most important aspects of digital imaging is the ability of the computer to mathematically change the image's brightness and contrast. Which of the following controls image brightness?

A. Window width
B. Window level
C. Digital filtering
D. Image resolution

B

549. RIS stands for:

A. Radiology information system
B. Rapid image sequence
C. Radiographic image system
D. Radiology image system

A

550. What does CCD stand for?

A. Capture-connection device
B. Charged-couple device
C. Computerized capturing device
D. Computer charging device

B

551. Which of the following is a logic function?

A. If .... then
B. Multiplication
C. Addition
D. Subtraction

A

552. Which of the following is a step-by-step procedure for solving a problem or accomplishing a task?

A. Subtraction
B. Calculation
C. Algorithm
D. Compiling

C

553. Visually, dynamic range refers to which of the following?

A. The number of shades of gray that can be represented
B. The number of pixels in a matrix
C. The range of numbers in a computer's memory
D. The size of the area of an image intensifier tube

A

554. PACS stands for:

A. pictures accessed by computers
B. picture archiving and communication system
C. patient access computer system
D. picture access computer system

B

555. Random background interference that is often referred to as "snow" on a television is called what?

A. Static
B. Signal ratio
C. Frequency
D. Noise

D

556. Which of the following refers to adding text to a digital image?

A. Verbalize
B. Delete
C. Work list
D. Annotate

D

557. In digital subtraction, which image is usually used for the mask?

A. The first image
B. The image right before the contrast appears
C. The image right after the contrast appears
D. The last image

B

558. Which of the following is an advantage of digital imaging over conventional imaging?

A. Less exposure time
B. Less noise
C. More resolution
D. More exposure latitude

D

559. The minimum matrix size for an acceptable digital radiographic image is which of the following?

A. 256 x 256
B. 512 x 512
C. 1024 x 1024
D. 2048 x 2048

C

560. What is the technical name for a computed radiography imaging plate?

A. PSL
B. CR cassette
C. Photostimulable phosphor plate - PSP
D. Photosensitive photon absorber

C

561. What does the CR reader use to release the energy stored in the image plate?

A. Red laser light
B. Infrared heat
C. Photomultiplier
D. Green visible light

A

562. Which of the following is a disadvantage of computed radiography (CR)?

A. Speed
B. Contrast
C. Resolution
D. Latitude

C

563. The amount of exposure required for CR is similar to which of the following film-screen systems?

A. 100 speed
B. 200 speed
C. 400 speed
D. 800 speed

B

564. An insufficient amount of mAs will produce a digital image with:

A. distortion.
B. loss of contrast.
C. noise.
D. loss of brightness.

C

565. Density was the term used to describe the overall blackening of a conventional radiograph. What term is used in digital radiography to describe this radiographic quality?

A. Window width
B. Exposure
C. Contrast
D. Brightness

D

566. Most computed radiography (CR) readers scan the image plate at what frequency?

A. 1000 x 1000
B. 2000 x 2000
C. 3000 x 3000
D. 4000 x 4000

B

567. What is the spatial resolution of a 24 cm x 30 cm (10 x 12) image plate?

A. 2 lp/mm
B. 3 lp/mm
C. 4 lp/mm
D. 5 lp/mm

C

568. Which of the following cassette-based imaging plates should be selected to produce an image with the best spatial resolution?

A. 18 cm x 24 cm (8 x 10)
B. 24 cm x 30 cm (10 x 12)
C. 30 cm x 35 cm (11 x 14)
D. 35 cm x 43 cm (14 x 17)

A

569. To prevent a moire pattern in your computed radiography (CR) digital image, it is best to have the grid lines running _____ to the direction of the laser beam.

A. perpendicular
B. diagonal
C. parallel
D. oblique

A

570. One image per image plate is preferred. Which of the following must be done to assure ideal processing of the image?

1. The exposure field is centered to the cassette
2. The anatomical part is centered to the cassette
3. Four collimated borders can be recognized

A. 1 only
B. 2 only
C. 2 & 3 only
D. 1, 2 & 3

D

571. Which of the following is true?

A. Low numbers represent low exposure, which will be light in the image.
B. Low numbers represent low exposure, which will be dark in the image.
C. Low numbers represent high exposure, which will be light in the image.
D. Low numbers represent high exposure, which will be dark in the image.

A

572. After the values of interest have been determined from the histogram, which of the following is used to automatically rescale those numbers to produce the proper contrast?

A. Contrast chart
B. Look-up table
C. Values graph
D. Numbers diagram

B

573. In order for the computer to accurately locate the appropriate anatomy, the part must be centered to the cassette and at least ______ sides of collimation detected.

A. 1
B. 2
C. 3
D. 4

C

574. Which of the following is least sensitive to low levels of radiation?

A. Film-screen
B. Cassette-based storage phosphors
C. Cassette-less detectors
D. Charge-coupled devices

A

575. A cassette-based imaging plate requires _____ of exposure to produce an optimum quality image.

A. 0.5 mR
B. 1.0 mR
C. 2.0 mR
D. 5.0 mR

B

576. With cassette-based systems, the exposure index is determined from the histogram. Which of the following could cause an incorrect value?

1. Anatomical part not centered to the cassette
2. Three sides of collimation not detected
3. Incorrect anatomical part selected from the menu

A. 1 only
B. 1 & 2 only
C. 2 & 3 only
D. 1, 2 & 3

D

577. Dose Area Product (DAP) is defined by which of the following?

A. The multiplication of the dose and the area exposed
B. The dose to an area surrounding the part
C. The larger the area the greater the dose
D. The product of time, distance and shielding

A

578. The histogram is used to automatically rescale the image to the proper brightness. Which of the following could cause an error with the histogram analysis?

1. Exposure field not detected
2. Unexpected metal in the data set
3. Gross overexposure

A. 1 & 2 only
B. 1 & 3 only
C. 2 & 3 only
D. 1, 2 & 3

D

579. Which of the following occurs when the imaging plate or detector is grossly overexposed?

A. Saturation
B. Intensification
C. Dynamic quantum
D. Dynamic inefficiency

A

580. Background radiation is approximately 40 microRoentgens - 80 microRoentgens per day. Cassette-based imaging plates are sensitive to levels of radiation as low as 60 microRoentgens. What is the rule for erasing the fog, caused by the background radiation, from the imaging plate?

A. Erase the imaging plate before each use
B. Erase the imaging plate once each morning
C. Erase the imaging plate if it has been unused for more than 48 hours
D. Erasing the imaging plate is not necessary since the background radiation levels are so low

C

581. How will grid cutoff appear on a digital image?

A. Low contrast and noise
B. High contrast and noise
C. Too bright
D. Too dark

A

582. Short dimension grids, where the grid lines run with the short axis of the grid instead of the normal long axis, are useful for which of the following?

A. Upright abdomen
B. Portable (mobile) chest done with the grid crosswise
C. Portable (mobile) knee in traction
D. 45/45 trauma shoulder

B

583. In digital radiography, Nyquist is referring to which of the following?

A. The efficiency of the flat-panel detector
B. The accuracy of the histogram
C. The sampling frequency of the digital data
D. The brightness of the laser beam

C

584. If the Nyquist frequency and the grid frequency are approximately the same, which of the following may occur?

A. Histogram error
B. Moire effect
C. Grid cutoff
D. Dark image

B

585. Smoothing can be applied to a digital image to mask which of the following?

A. Artifacts
B. Metal objects
C. Fog
D. Noise

D

586. Edge enhancement can be applied to a digital image to improve which of the following?

A. The black border around the edge of the image
B. The loss of details in the image
C. The contrast along the edges of a structure
D. The sharpness of structural lines

C

587. Applying too much edge enhancement to a digital image can result in which of the following?

A. Loss of visibility of details
B. Halo artifact
C. Noise
D. Loss of recorded details

B

588. Noise in low exposure areas and saturation in high exposure areas can result when which one of the following post processing techniques is excessively applied?

A. Window level
B. Smoothing
C. Edge enhancement
D. Equalization

D

589. How can the radiographer tell if the automatic exposure control (AEC) is calibrated properly when using cassette-based digital systems?

A. Window level adjustments are not necessary
B. Compare the histogram to the look-up table
C. The exposure indicator number is in the optimal range
D. Calculate the pixel values

C

590. Which of the following can be used to reduce patient exposure since cassette-based digital systems require more exposure than film-screen systems?

1. Use higher kVp
2. Increase beam filtration
3. Use automatic exposure control (AEC)

A. 1 & 2 only
B. 1 & 3 only
C. 2 & 3 only
D. 1, 2 & 3

D

591. Thin film transistors (TFT) are found in which type of digital system?

A. Computed radiography
B. Cassette-less
C. Cassette-based
D. CCD

B

592. _______ phosphors are randomly suspended in the phosphor layer, whereas, _____ phosphors are grown into columns.

A. Stored, fixed
B. Photostimulable, plate
C. Turbid, structured
D. Europium, barium fluoride

C

593. The latent image can remain "stored" in the photostimulable phosphor (PSP) plate for _____ hours before information is lost.

A. 8
B. 16
C. 24
D. 36

A

594. A cassette-less system's detector element (DEL) size determines which of the following?

A. Dynamic range
B. Detective quantum efficiency (DQE)
C. Pixel size
D. Speed class

C

595. Contrast resolution is a major advantage of digital imaging. What determines high contrast resolution in a digital image?

A. High exposure and low noise
B. Low exposure and high noise
C. High exposure and high resolution
D. High resolution and low noise

A

596. Presently, cassette-less systems do not have exposure indicators. Which of the following can determine if the proper exposure was made?

A. Multiply mAs x kVp
B. Measure the Dose Area Product (DAP)
C. Analyze the background fog
D. Calculate the size of the area x centimeter thickness

B

597. A flat-panel detector requires ____ of exposure to produce an optimum quality image.

A. 0.5 mR
B. 1.0 mR
C. 2.0 mR
D. 5.0 mR

A

598. When the computers in a hospital are connected together you have a _____.

A. DICOM
B. WAN
C. LAN
D. VPN

C

599. Which of the following is necessary to connect a computer outside of the hospital to the hospital's server?

A. WAN
B. LAN
C. VPN
D. FOV

C

600. The three-dimensional volume of tissue that is represented in each pixel is known as what?

A. 3D space
B. Tissue volume
C. A voxel
D. A matrix

C

601. The size of the pixel produced when a cassette-based imaging plate is read depends on which of the following?

1. The speed of the imaging plate as it passes through the reader
2. The frequency with which the data is sampled
3. The dimensions of the laser beam

A. 1 only
B. 1 & 2 only
C. 1 & 3 only
D. 1, 2 & 3

D

602. Which of the following would NOT be part of a direct capture flat-panel detector?

A. Glass substrate
B. Fluorescent layer
C. TFT layer
D. Photoconductor layer

B

603. With digital imaging, brightness and contrast are almost always acceptable. Which of the following would cause a digital image to display low contrast?

A. Improper kVp used
B. Exposure time too short
C. Overexposure of the imaging plate by 4X
D. Underexposure of the imaging plate by 4X

C

604. There are direct and indirect ways of capturing an x-ray image with cassette-less digital systems. Arrange the following in the order they are layered, from top to bottom, in an indirect flat-panel detector.

1. Photodetector layer
2. Fluorescent layer
3. TFT layer

A. 1, 2, then 3
B. 1, 3, then 2
C. 2, 1, then 3
D. 3, 2, then 1

C

605. Extreme overexposure (at least 4X) will create "black holes" in the low density, tissue areas of a digital image. The proper term for this effect is:

A. noise.
B. saturation.
C. pixel drop.
D. quasar.

B

606. Which of the following could cause a histogram analysis error?

1. Improper collimation
2. Off focus/scatter radiation
3. Grid cut-off

A. 1 & 2 only
B. 1 & 3 only
C. 2 & 3 only
D. 1, 2 & 3

D

607. How would dirt in the light guide of a CR reader appear on a digital image?

A. White lines
B. Black lines
C. Gray lines
D. Dark gray lines

A

608. Which of the following initial acceptance tests should be done on digital detectors before the final payment is made?

1. Test for dark noise
2. Test for uniformity
3. Test for erasure thoroughness

A. 1 & 2 only
B. 1 & 3 only
C. 2 & 3 only
D. 1, 2 & 3

D

609. A quality assurance test for digital imaging receptors is to check for dark noise. What is the purpose of this test?

A. To determine the maximum exposure that can be detected
B. To listen for static in the reader
C. To assess the level of detector noise in the system
D. To evaluate the monitor's window level settings

C

610. Which of the following should be part of initial acceptance testing of a CR reader?

1. Uniformity of image receptors
2. Erasure thoroughness
3. Reader calibration

A. 1 & 2 only
B. 1 & 3 only
C. 2 & 3 only
D. 1, 2 & 3

D

611. ______ releases electrons when struck by light photons and ______ releases electrons when struck by x ray photons.

A. Gadolinium oxysulfide, cesium iodide
B. Amorphous silicon, amorphous selenium
C. Amorphous selenium, amorphous silicon
D. Silver bromide, zinc lead sulfide

B

612. Which of the following is true concerning indirect digital radiography compared to direct digital radiography?

A. Less exposure to the patient and less resolution
B. Less exposure to the patient and more resolution
C. More exposure to the patient and less resolution
D. More exposure to the patient and more resolution

A

613. What is the definition of amorphous?

A. A noncrystalline state of an otherwise crystalline material
B. The process of emitting light when stimulated by x rays
C. Converting x rays to light
D. Storing electrical charge for digital viewing

A

CHAPTER THREE

IMAGE PRODUCTION

- Radiographic Accessories (70 questions)
- Processing (56 questions)
- Recorded Detail (44 questions)
- Distortion (30 questions)
- Density (36 questions)
- Contrast (46 questions)
- Technique Problems (42 questions)

RADIOGRAPHIC ACCESSORIES

614. The front of a cassette can be made from which of the following materials?

1. Bakelite
2. Aluminum
3. Plastic

A. 1 only
B. 3 only
C. 2 & 3 only
D. 1, 2 & 3

D

615. What is the color of light emitted by a gadolinium oxysulfide rare earth intensifying screen?

A. Amber
B. Blue
C. Green
D. White

C

616. The major difference between a 200 speed screen and a 400 speed screen is which of the following?

A. Size of phosphor
B. Shape of phosphor
C. Thickness of phosphor layer
D. Color of reflective paint

C

617. An illuminator (viewbox) should have a fluorescent bulb with how much light intensity?

A. 1500 NIT
B. 2500 NIT
C. 3500 NIT
D. 4500 NIT

A

618. An unexposed radiographic film will have a slight density after processing. What is this density called?

A. Fog
B. Base plus fog
C. Base density
D. Gamma

B

619. Which of the following materials would NOT be used in the interspaces of a grid?

A. Aluminum
B. Fiber (cardboard)
C. Polyester plastic
D. Lead

D

620. When should a grid be used?

1. When radiographing body parts greater than 10 cm
2. When using high kVp
3. When scatter radiation is high

A. 1 & 2 only
B. 1 & 3 only
C. 2 & 3 only
D. 1, 2 & 3

D

621. What is a major benefit of a fixed kVp technique chart?

A. Consistent radiographic contrast
B. Decreased exposure latitude
C. Increased tube loading
D. Increase in patient exposure

A

622. Which of the following is the main determinant in selecting a focal spot size?

A. The kVp used
B. The mA used
C. The equipment manufacturer
D. The SID

B

623. Compared to a low ratio grid, a high ratio grid will do which of the following?

A. Absorb more primary radiation
B. Absorb more scatter radiation
C. Absorb less primary radiation
D. Absorb less scatter radiation

B

624. When using a tube rating chart, which of the following must be taken into consideration?

1. Focal spot size
2. Speed of rotor
3. Size of generator

A. 1 only
B. 1 & 2 only
C. 2 & 3 only
D. 1, 2 & 3

B

625. How can a compression band improve radiographic quality?

1. Reduce scatter radiation
2. Reduce patient motion
3. Improve radiographic contrast

A. 1 only
B. 2 only
C. 1 & 3 only
D. 1, 2 & 3

D

626. Which of the following tests will determine the focal spot size?

A. Safelight test
B. Wire mesh test
C. Wisconsin test cassette
D. Star pattern test

D

627. Off-distance grid cut-off is characterized by which of the following?

A. The top of the image is underexposed
B. Both sides of the image are underexposed
C. One side of the image is underexposed
D. The bottom of the image is underexposed

B

628. What is the main reason why beam filters are used in radiography?

A. Improves contrast
B. Improves radiographic quality
C. Reduces patient exposure
D. Prolongs tube life

C

629. What is a 3-dimensional radiograph called that is produced by two angled views of the same structure?

A. Stereoradiograph
B. Tomogram
C. Scanogram
D. Bi-radiograph

A

630. The use of intensifying screens will have which of the following effects?

A. Decrease patient exposure
B. Decrease contrast
C. Decrease density
D. Decrease radiographic fog

A

631. What does it mean if a radiographic film is duplitized?

A. Twice as dense
B. Twice as thick
C. Developed two times
D. Emulsion is coated on two sides

D

632. Which of the following is an example of a compensating filter?

A. Inherent filter
B. Added filter
C. Aluminum wedge filter
D. Collimator

C

633. How can the production of scatter radiation be reduced?

1. Increase kVp
2. Use close collimation
3. Increase beam filtration

A. 1 only
B. 2 only
C. 1 & 3 only
D. 1, 2 & 3

B

634. Which of the following is used to reduce the effect of scatter radiation?

A. Intensifying screens
B. Compensating filters
C. Radiographic grids
D. Compression devices

C

635. Which of the following is found in the emulsion of radiographic film?

A. Silver bromide
B. Silver nitrate
C. Potassium bromide
D. Calcium tungstate

A

636. The emulsion on a radiographic film is composed of silver halide crystals suspended in _____.

A. Polyester
B. Plastic
C. Cellulose
D. Gelatin

D

637. What is it called when an intensifying screen continues to fluoresce after the exposure is completed?

A. Luminescence
B. Fluorescence
C. Phosphorescence
D. Incandescence

C

638. How much should kVp be increased when an extension cylinder is used to cone down on an area of interest?

A. 5 kVp
B. 10 kVp
C. 15 kVp
D. 20 kVp

A

639. Which of the following materials is classified as a rare earth phosphor?

A. Calcium tungstate
B. Gadolinium oxysulfide
C. Silver bromide
D. Lead barium sulfate

B

640. Exposure required without screens divided by exposure required with screens defines which of the following?

A. Intensification factor
B. Reciprocity ratio
C. Image intensification
D. Resolving ratio

A

641. Poor film-screen contact can be caused by which of the following?

1. Warped cassette front
2. Bent cassette frame
3. Broken cassette latch

A. 1 & 2 only
B. 1 & 3 only
C. 2 & 3 only
D. 1, 2 & 3

D

642. Which of the following is the least acceptable beam restricting device?

A. Collimator
B. Diaphragm
C. Cone
D. Cylinder

B

643. The base of radiographic film is made from which of the following materials?

A. Glass
B. Cellulose acetate
C. Polyester plastic
D. Cardboard

C

644. 400 speed rare earth screens require how much less radiation than 200 speed rare earth screens?

A. 25% less
B. 50% less
C. 100% less
D. 200% less

B

645. The image on radiographic film after exposure but before development is known as what?

A. A latent image
B. A manifest image
C. A visible image
D. An imaginary image

A

646. Radiographic quality is achieved by balancing which of the following?

A. Density and contrast
B. Recorded detail and distortion
C. Sharpness of detail and visibility of detail
D. Recorded detail and contrast

C

647. Off-center grid cut-off would demonstrate which of these?

A. The top of the image would be underexposed
B. One side of the image would be underexposed
C. Both sides of the image would be underexposed
D. The bottom of the image would be underexposed

B

648. A characteristic curve graphically demonstrates the relationship between which of the following?

A. Density and contrast
B. Detail and distortion
C. Density and exposure
D. Contrast and exposure

C

649. Which of the following is NOT a primary factor in the production of a radiograph?

A. mA
B. Seconds
C. kVp
D. Intensification factor

D

650. What is the purpose of a compensating filter?

A. Reduce patient exposure
B. Reduce skin dose
C. Produce better detail in a radiograph
D. Produce uniform density in a radiograph

D

651. A fixed-kVp technique chart uses which of the following?

A. Fixed kVp and fixed mAs
B. Fixed kVp and variable mAs
C. Fixed mAs and variable kVp
D. Variable mAs and variable kVp

B

652. Why do the backs of some cassettes contain lead?

1. Stops backscatter from fogging the film
2. Stops scatter from striking the patient
3. Stops x rays from leaving the cassette

A. 1 only
B. 2 only
C. 1 & 3 only
D. 1, 2 & 3

A

653. Subtraction technique is used for which of the following situations?

A. Orthopedic studies
B. Gastrointestinal studies
C. Angiographic studies
D. Tomographic studies

C

654. Which of the following tests will determine film-screen contact?

A. Safelight test
B. Spinning top test
C. Acid test
D. Wire mesh test

D

655. Because of the anode heel effect, where is the intensity of the x-ray beam the greatest?

A. At the anode end
B. At the cathode end
C. At the rotor end
D. In the center of the beam

B

656. How many lines per inch are normal in modern radiographic grids?

A. 60
B. 80
C. 100
D. 120

C

657. A radiographic grid should be used whenever kVp exceeds which of the following?

A. 30 kVp
B. 40 kVp
C. 50 kVp
D. 60 kVp

D

658. Which of the following grid interspaces will produce the most satisfactory radiograph?

A. Fiber (cardboard)
B. Polyester
C. Plastic
D. Aluminum

D

659. Which of the following would NOT be classified as a beam restricting device?

A. Collimator
B. Port
C. Diaphragm
D. Cylinder

B

660. Which of the following causes the most repeated radiographs in a radiology department?

A. Motion
B. Positioning errors
C. Under and over exposed radiographs
D. Poor contrast

B

661. What is the function of a cassette?

A. Maintain good film-screen contact
B. Protect film from light
C. Protect film from backscatter
D. Protect film from x rays

A

662. Which of the following statements concerning a 16:1 ratio grid is true?

1. Effectively absorbs scatter rays
2. Designed for high kVp techniques
3. Has little positioning latitude

A. 1 only
B. 1 & 3 only
C. 2 & 3 only
D. 1, 2 & 3

D

663. A compression band will improve which of the following radiographic qualities?

A. Density
B. Contrast
C. Distortion
D. Recorded detail

B

664. Which of the four primary factors in the production of a radiograph is regarded as the factor of penetration?

A. mA
B. Seconds
C. kVp
D. SID

C

665. The height of the lead strips divided by the distance between the lead strips defines which of the following?

A. Grid ratio
B. Grid focusing distance
C. Grid frequency
D. Grid tolerance

A

666. Which of the following relates to the principle of light reflecting through the film base?

A. Line focus principle
B. Photoelectric absorption
C. Parallax effect
D. Characteristic effect

C

667. The rare earth phosphor, lanthanum oxybromide, emits what color light?

A. Amber
B. Green
C. Blue
D. White

C

668. What type of screen was present when Roentgen discovered x rays?

A. Calcium tungstate
B. Barium lead sulfate
C. Lanthanum oxybromide
D. Barium platinocyanide

D

669. A properly formulated technique chart could accurately be used for what percentage of patients?

A. 25%
B. 50%
C. 75%
D. 90%

D

670. What does grid cut-off mean?

A. The primary x rays are absorbed
B. The secondary x rays are absorbed
C. The scatter x rays are absorbed
D. The remnant (exit) x rays are absorbed

A

671. Which of the following conditions will cause grid cut-off with a focused grid?

1. CR not centered to grid
2. Grid angled
3. Tube angled across the grid

A. 1 only
B. 2 only
C. 2 & 3 only
D. 1, 2 & 3

D

672. Grid focusing distance is associated with which of the following?

A. Grid ratio
B. Lines per inch
C. Focused grids
D. Parallel grids

C

673. Quality assurance programs suggest radiographic illuminators (viewboxes) should be cleaned how often?

A. Daily
B. Weekly
C. Monthly
D. Yearly

C

674. Which type of radiographic grid has lead lines running in two directions?

A. Linear
B. Cross hatch
C. Parallel
D. Focused

B

675. The image on a radiograph after development is known as what?

A. A latent image
B. A manifest image
C. An invisible image
D. An imaginary image

B

676. What is it called when a phosphor absorbs x rays and immediately emits light?

A. Fluorescence
B. Brightescence
C. Phosphorescence
D. Incandescence

A

677. When mA is increased, what must be done to exposure time in order to maintain the same density?

A. Increase time
B. Decrease time
C. Keep the time the same
D. Match time with kVp

B

678. Where is the ionization chamber (photocell) located in an automatic exposure control (AEC) device?

A. Between the tube and the patient
B. Between the patient and the image receptor
C. Behind the image receptor
D. Below the Bucky tray

B

679. The distance between the lead strips of a focused grid to a point where all lines converge is known as what?

A. Grid ratio
B. Grid focusing distance
C. Grid frequency
D. Grid tolerance

B

680. Which of the following is an advantage of the air gap technique?

A. Easier to position the patient
B. Greater exposure latitude
C. Allows for a short SID
D. Eliminates the need for a grid

D

681. Teleroentgenography refers to any radiograph taken at what SID?

A. 36"
B. 40"
C. 60"
D. 72"

D

682. Which of the following affects grid efficiency the most?

A. Grid ratio
B. Grid focusing distance
C. Grid frequency
D. Grid tolerance

A

683. No practical amount of mAs can ever compensate for which of the following?

A. Inadequate exposure time
B. Inadequate kVp
C. Inadequate SID
D. Inadequate grid ratio

B

PROCESSING

684. Which of the following is the major cause of artifacts on a radiograph?

A. Improper handling of the film
B. Improper storage of the film
C. Outdated film
D. Incorrect techniques

A

685. Under what conditions should x-ray film be stored?

A. Warm, dry room
B. Warm, humid room
C. Cool, dry room
D. Cool, humid room

C

686. According to quality assurance programs, how often should the chemicals be changed in a processor?

A. Once a day
B. Once a week
C. Once a month
D. Once a year

C

687. Chemical fog on a radiograph results from which of the following?

A. Too high of a developer temperature
B. Too high of a fixer temperature
C. Too high of a dryer temperature
D. Too high of a water temperature

A

688. If the developer replenishment is set too low, which of the following will result?

1. Films will not fix or dry
2. Films will show low contrast
3. Films will be too dark

A. 1 only
B. 2 only
C. 3 only
D. 2 & 3 only

B

689. Which of the following will cause improper agitation in an automatic film processor?

A. Clogged replenishment line
B. Loose transport roller
C. Broken circulation pump
D. Low water pressure

C

690. Underreplenishment of the fixer in an automatic processor will result in which of the following problems?

A. Dirty films
B. Low contrast films
C. Chemical fog
D. Wet, sticky films

D

691. Which of the following types of film will require a sheet of leader film to guide it through the processor?

A. Polaroid film
B. Roll film
C. Mammography film
D. CT film

B

692. Which of the following will have the greatest effect on causing the processor to go "out of control"?

A. Fluctuation in developer temperature
B. Increased replenishment rates
C. Amount of water flow
D. Dryer temperature too low

A

693. Which of the following should be checked during the day in order to assure quality film processing?

1. Replenishment rates
2. Hypo retention
3. Developer temperatures

A. 1 only
B. 3 only
C. 2 & 3 only
D. 1, 2 & 3

B

694. Which chemical in the developer causes the film emulsion to swell?

A. Potassium bromide
B. Sodium sulfite
C. Hydroquinone
D. Sodium carbonate

D

695. What happens to developer if it is exposed to the air for a long period of time?

A. It becomes contaminated
B. It becomes oxidized
C. It becomes a milky color
D. It becomes fixer

B

696. Why does the manufacturer seal x-ray film in plastic containers?

A. To prevent static
B. To protect it from moisture
C. To eliminate the risk of radiation fog
D. To keep film clean

B

697. Low humidity in the darkroom can cause which of the following artifacts?

A. Static
B. Crinkle marks
C. Quantum Mottle
D. Reticulation

A

698. Developer temperatures in 90 second automatic processors fall in which of the following ranges?

A. 60-65^0 Fahrenheit
B. 70-75^0 Fahrenheit
C. 80-85^0 Fahrenheit
D. 90-95^0 Fahrenheit

D

699. Reducing agents convert silver halide crystals into which of the following?

A. Potassium bromide
B. Silver nitrate
C. Black metallic silver
D. Sensitivity specks

C

700. Which of the following prevents the developer from reducing unexposed silver bromide crystals?

A. Activator
B. Restrainer
C. Solvent
D. Preservative

B

701. What is the purpose of the fixer in an automatic processor?

A. Reduce the exposed silver halide crystals
B. Remove the unexposed silver halide crystals
C. Remove the emulsion
D. Harden the base

B

702. Which of the following is true concerning the unexposed silver halide crystals?

1. They are unaffected by the developer
2. They are removed by the fixer
3. They represent the latent image

A. 1 only
B. 1 & 2 only
C. 2 & 3 only
D. 1, 2 & 3

B

703. Which of the following would be considered the most important factor in the developing process?

A. The temperature of the developer
B. The amount of developer
C. The number of films developed
D. The brand of developer

A

704. Sodium sulfite is found in both the developer and fixer. What is its purpose?

A. Activator
B. Solvent
C. Preservative
D. Hardener

C

705. Which of the following converts the invisible latent image into a visible manifest image?

A. Reducer
B. Activator
C. Preservative
D. Hardener

A

706. When is x-ray film most sensitive to safelight illumination?

A. Before exposure
B. After exposure
C. When humidity is high
D. When temperatures are high

B

707. Where would the expiration date for radiographic film be found?

A. On the inside cover of the box
B. On each individual film
C. On each individual box of film
D. This data is kept by the manufacturer

C

708. Which of the following is necessary while handling radiographic film?

1. Hands must be clean and dry
2. Move film rapidly
3. Handle film only in the center

A. 1 only
B. 1 & 3 only
C. 2 & 3 only
D. 1, 2 & 3

A

709. Which of the following best describes the fixer solution?

A. Weak alkali
B. Weak acid
C. Weak solution
D. Neutral solution

B

710. Which of the following is NOT necessary for proper quality control of the processor?

A. Accurate replenishment rates
B. Accurate solution temperatures
C. Accurate silver recovery
D. Accurate time of processing

C

711. Which of the following is the correct automatic processing cycle?

A. Develop, fix, wash, dry
B. Develop, wash, fix, dry
C. Develop, fix, dry, wash
D. Develop, wash, fix, wash

A

712. A silver recovery unit attached to the processor can result in which of the following?

A. Conserve developer
B. Conserve fixer
C. Conserve energy
D. Conserve money

D

713. Which of the following is usually the cause of the films coming out of the processor wet and sticky?

A. Exhausted developer
B. Exhausted fixer
C. Wash water pressure too low
D. Wash water temperature too low

B

714. A well organized quality control program will assure which of the following?

1. Minimal exposure to patients
2. Consistent radiographic quality
3. Minimum down-time of equipment

A. 1 & 2 only
B. 1 & 3 only
C. 2 & 3 only
D. 1, 2 & 3

D

715. Which of the following chemicals would be found only in the fixer?

A. Hydroquinone
B. Potassium bromide
C. Potassium alum
D. Sodium sulfite

C

716. Which of the following chemicals found in the fixer is the clearing agent?

A. Sodium sulfite
B. Potassium alum
C. Acetic acid
D. Ammonium thiosulfate

D

717. What type of filter is used in darkroom safelights to produce a dark red illumination?

A. Kodak GBX
B. Kodak DRX
C. Kodak wratten 6B
D. Kodak wratten 8B

A

718. What could be the cause of excessive density throughout the radiographic film?

A. Overdevelopment
B. Underexposure
C. Prolonged fixation
D. Too low of a developer temperature

A

719. What might cause small, white marks on a finished radiograph?

A. Rapid movement of exposed film
B. Dirty screens
C. Low water pressure
D. Exhausted developer

B

720. What is the function of the preservative in the developer and the fixer?

1. Prevent overdevelopment and fixation
2. Prolong the life of the solutions
3. Preserve the finished radiograph

A. 1 only
B. 2 only
C. 3 only
D. 1 & 2 only

B

721. A spotty, salt and pepper effect on a radiograph caused by low levels of radiation intensity is called what?

A. Penumbra
B. Safelight fog
C. Quantum mottle
D. Chemical fog

C

722. Which of the following is an advantage of automatic film processing?

A. Less costly
B. No need for darkroom technicians
C. Consistent radiographic quality
D. Standardized development

D

723. Outdated film may show which of the following problems?

A. Loss of contrast
B. Green emulsion
C. Reticulation
D. Inability to dry

A

724. How high above the working area should a safelight be installed?

A. 12"
B. 24"
C. 36"
D. 48"

C

725. How will an increase in developer temperature from 90^0-95^0F affect the radiographic image?

A. Decrease contrast
B. Decrease density
C. Increase density
D. Increase distortion

C

726. If a film is fogged, which of the following could have caused the problem?

1. A light leak
2. Contaminated developer
3. Exhausted developer

A. 1 & 2 only
B. 1 & 3 only
C. 2 & 3 only
D. 1, 2 & 3

D

727. What is the most likely cause of contaminated developer?

A. Overreplenishment
B. Underreplenishment
C. Developing too many films
D. Fixer being splashed into developer

D

728. Which of the following artifacts may result if a radiographic film is bent?

A. Quantum mottle
B. Tree static
C. Crinkle mark
D. Crown static

C

729. Covering half of an exposed film while it is lying on the darkroom bench and then processing it describes what?

A. Film-screen contact test
B. Safelight test
C. Radiographic film test
D. Processing test

B

730. If two films are run through the processor at the same time, what will be the result?

A. Only the top film will be processed
B. The bottom film will be clear
C. Both films will be normal
D. The inner surfaces will be unprocessed

D

731. If the wash water is not turned on, or the water pressure is too low, what will the radiograph look like?

A. Greasy appearance
B. Underdeveloped
C. Surface will be wet
D. Film will lack contrast

A

732. If safelight filter and distance are correct, what size bulb should be used?

A. 5-7 watt
B. 10-15 watt
C. 20-25 watt
D. 30 watt

B

733. Anything that is foreign to the normal radiographic image is called what?

A. An artifact
B. A blemish
C. A foreign body
D. "*&/$#@%"

A

734. Which of the following types of static is caused by pulling the film from the film bin too rapidly?

A. Tree static
B. Smudge static
C. Crown static
D. Branch static

C

735. Which of the following types of static is caused by removing the film from the cassette too rapidly?

A. Tree static
B. Smudge static
C. Crown static
D. Proton static

A

736. Equally spaced scratches at the leading and trailing edges of a film are caused by which of these?

A. Dirty rollers
B. A guide shoe
C. A slipping roller
D. Weak fixer

B

737. What is the name of the rollers in the processor that reduce the amount of carry-over of solutions?

A. Entrance rollers
B. Transport rollers
C. Squeegee rollers
D. Dryer rollers

C

738. Scratches that are equally spaced about 3.14" apart are called what?

A. Pi lines
B. Guide shoe lines
C. Plus density lines
D. Smudge lines

A

739. Which of the following is NOT a system of an automatic processor?

A. Transport
B. Replenishment
C. Chemistry
D. Filtering

D

RECORDED DETAIL

740. A decrease in exposure time may increase which of the following?

A. Density
B. Contrast
C. Distortion
D. Recorded detail

D

741. What is the definition of recorded detail?

A. The contrast in the image
B. The sharpness of the structural lines
C. The lack of distortion in the image
D. All of the above are good definitions

B

742. Loss of recorded detail due to the use of intensifying screens is referred to as what?

A. Intrinsic unsharpness
B. Distortion
C. Gamma loss
D. Detail loss

A

743. Which of the following screen speeds will produce the best recorded detail?

A. 50
B. 100
C. 200
D. 400

A

744. Which of the following factors is unrelated to recorded detail?

A. Geometric factors
B. Motion factors
C. Intrinsic factors
D. Technical factors of kVp and mA

D

745. Recorded detail can be improved by which of the following?

A. Higher contrast
B. Greater density
C. Smaller focal spot size
D. Air gap technique

C

746. Recorded detail can be improved by which of the following?

A. Maximum OID
B. Maximum SID
C. Minimum SID
D. Minimum SOD

B

747. What is the correct name for the loss of recorded detail due to the use of large focal spots or intensifying screens?

A. Umbra
B. Mottle
C. Blur
D. Unsharpness

D

748. The ability of a system to record detail (expressed as the number of line pairs per millimeter) is known as its what?

A. Resolving power
B. Quality assurance
C. Detail factor
D. Finite factor

A

749. Poor film-screen contact will cause which of the following effects?

A. Gain of contrast
B. Unsharpness
C. Loss of density
D. Gain of recorded detail

B

750. Which of the following could be the cause of poor film-screen contact?

1. Warped cassette
2. Worn backing in the cassette
3. Damaged latch on the cassette

A. 1 only
B. 3 only
C. 2 & 3 only
D. 1, 2 & 3

D

751. Which of the following intrinsic factors will have the greatest effect on recorded detail?

A. Screen speed
B. Film-screen contact
C. X-ray film
D. Size of image receptor

B

752. Which of the following is NOT considered one of the geometric factors that control recorded detail?

A. OID
B. SID
C. Focal spot size
D. Size of the object

D

753. Which of the following is the single most important reason for the loss of recorded detail in a radiograph?

A. Focal spot size
B. OID
C. Patient motion
D. Screen speed

B

754. Which of the following factors has the least effect on recorded detail?

A. Patient motion
B. Patient size
C. Focal spot size
D. Screen speed

B

755. Unsharpness is NOT affected by which of the following?

A. SID
B. SOD
C. OID
D. kVp

D

756. Patient motion can be used to an advantage in which of the following procedures?

A. Chest radiography
B. Coronary angiography
C. Lateral thoracic spine
D. Gastrointestinal radiography

C

757. When radiographing a small part, recorded detail can be improved by which of the following?

A. Using slow speed screens
B. Increasing the OID
C. Using a large focal spot
D. Using the high speed rotor

A

758. Which of the following will decrease the recorded detail in a radiograph?

1. Increasing the focal spot
2. Increasing screen speed
3. Increasing OID

A. 1 only
B. 2 only
C. 1 & 3 only
D. 1, 2 & 3

D

759. Which of the following refers to the amount of recorded detail on a radiograph?

A. Latitude
B. Gamma
C. Resolution
D. Exposure

C

760. Geometric unsharpness is directly proportional to which of the following?

1. SID
2. OID
3. SOD

A. 1 only
B. 2 only
C. 1 & 3 only
D. 1, 2 & 3

B

761. Which of the primary factors will always have an effect on recorded detail?

A. Seconds
B. SID
C. mA
D. kVp

B

762. Which of the following types of motion must be considered when setting a radiographic technique?

1. Voluntary
2. Involuntary
3. Accidental

A. 1 only
B. 1 & 2 only
C. 2 & 3 only
D. 1, 2 & 3

D

763. Recorded detail can be improved by reducing which of the following?

A. SID
B. SOD
C. Focal spot size
D. Patient size

C

764. Which of the following factors is the best for reducing the risks of motion?

A. High speed screens
B. Shortest possible exposure time
C. Low ratio grid
D. Highest practical kVp

D

765. Recorded detail is affected by which of the following?

A. Grid ratio
B. kVp
C. Filtration
D. Screen speed

D

766. Which of the following radiographic qualities determines the sharpness of detail in the finished radiograph?

A. Recorded detail and contrast
B. Recorded detail and distortion
C. Density and contrast
D. Density and distortion

B

767. In order to obtain the most recorded detail, the OID should be what?

A. The same for every image
B. As long as possible
C. As short as possible
D. Equal to the SID

C

768. Which of the following may be used to control motion during a radiographic examination?

1. Immobilization devices
2. Precise verbal instructions to the patient
3. Shortest possible exposure time

A. 1 only
B. 1 & 3 only
C. 2 & 3 only
D. 1, 2 & 3

D

769. If it is impossible to get the part close to the image receptor, what can be done to compensate?

A. Increase exposure time
B. Increase SID
C. Decrease kVp
D. Decrease screen speed

B

770. Which of the following will improve recorded detail?

A. Increase focal spot size
B. Increase filtration
C. Decrease field size
D. Decrease screen speed

D

771. Which of the following does NOT have any effect on recorded detail?

A. X-ray film
B. Grid ratio
C. Screen speed
D. Focal spot size

B

772. How will increasing the focal spot size affect recorded detail?

A. It will decrease blur
B. It will decrease unsharpness
C. It will increase unsharpness
D. It will increase recorded detail

C

773. How well an imaging system reproduces the sharpness of the actual object is referred to as what?

A. Modulation transfer function
B. Resolving power
C. Lines per inch
D. Linear image transfer

A

774. Which of the following methods can be used to control motion by reducing exposure time?

1. Use highest mA station possible
2. Increase kVp
3. Decrease SID

A. 1 only
B. 1 & 2 only
C. 1 & 3 only
D. 1, 2 & 3

D

775. Which of the following will probably have the greatest effect on reducing motion on an abdomen radiograph?

A. Suspend respiration
B. Compression device
C. High mA
D. Increased SID

A

776. For single-phase equipment, when motion is a problem, time can be reduced by 1/2 if the kVp is increased by what percentage?

A. 5%
B. 15%
C. 25%
D. 35%

B

777. The loss of recorded detail due to the materials used to make the screens and film is called what?

A. Fog
B. Detail loss
C. Intrinsic unsharpness
D. Distortion

C

778. How will increasing the OID affect the recorded detail in a radiograph?

A. Increase recorded detail
B. Decrease recorded detail
C. Eliminate recorded detail
D. Will have no effect on recorded detail

B

779. How will increasing the focal spot size affect the recorded detail in a radiograph?

A. Increase recorded detail
B. Decrease recorded detail
C. Eliminate recorded detail
D. Will have no effect on recorded detail

B

780. Which of the following can be used to reduce unsharpness?

1. Decrease screen speed
2. Decrease focal spot size
3. Decrease OID

A. 1 & 2 only
B. 1 & 3 only
C. 2 & 3 only
D. 1, 2 & 3

D

781. How will increasing SID affect the recorded detail in a radiograph?

A. Increase recorded detail
B. Decrease recorded detail
C. Eliminate recorded detail
D. Will have no effect on recorded detail

A

782. How will increasing screen speed affect the recorded detail in a radiograph?

A. Increase recorded detail
B. Decrease recorded detail
C. Eliminate recorded detail
D. Will have no effect on recorded detail

B

783. How will increasing film-screen contact affect the recorded detail on a radiograph?

A. Increase recorded detail
B. Decrease recorded detail
C. Eliminate recorded detail
D. Will have no effect on recorded detail

A

DISTORTION

784. Misrepresentation of the true size or shape of an object is the definition of which of the following?

A. Recorded detail
B. Elongation
C. Distortion
D. Magnification

C

785. What are the two types of distortion that can reduce the quality of a radiograph?

A. Size and shape
B. Size and contrast
C. Density and contrast
D. Long and short

A

786. Which of the following is the most important factor in controlling size distortion?

A. Focal spot size
B. SID
C. OID
D. Exposure time

C

787. Which of the following will keep size distortion to a minimum?

A. Increase screen speed
B. Increase grid ratio
C. Increase SID
D. Increase focal spot size

C

788. Which of the following occurs when the OID is increased?

A. Image size is reduced
B. Image is magnified
C. Image is elongated
D. Image is foreshortened

B

789. Which of the following distances would produce the least distortion?

1. 40"
2. 72"
3. Teleroentgen distance

A. 1 only
B. 1 & 3 only
C. 2 & 3 only
D. 1, 2 & 3

C

790. Size distortion can be used to an advantage for which of the following radiographic procedures?

A. Gastrointestinal
B. Skeletal
C. Angiographic
D. Neurological

C

791. Tube angulation will produce which of the following types of shape distortion?

A. Elongation
B. Foreshortening
C. Magnification
D. Minification

A

792. The ratio of SID to SOD represents which of the following?

A. Distortion ratio
B. Magnification ratio
C. Definition ratio
D. Shape ratio

B

793. When an object is placed halfway between the tube and the image receptor the image will be how many times larger?

A. 2X
B. 3X
C. 4X
D. 8X

A

794. Which of the following focal spot sizes should be used when doing macro radiography?

A. .3 mm
B. 1.0 mm
C. 1.5 mm
D. 2.0 mm

A

795. What percentage increase is usually used for magnification radiography?

A. 25%
B. 50%
C. 75%
D. 100%

D

796. Which of the following would be used to minimize size distortion?

1. Shortest possible OID
2. Smallest focal spot size
3. Longest SID

A. 1 only
B. 1 & 3 only
C. 2 & 3 only
D. 1, 2 & 3

B

797. What type of distortion results from an increase in OID?

A. Minification
B. Size
C. Elongation
D. Shape

B

798. A misrepresentation of the shape of an object may be caused by which of the following?

1. An angled object
2. An angled x-ray tube
3. An angled image receptor

A. 1 & 2 only
B. 1 & 3 only
C. 2 & 3 only
D. 1, 2 & 3

D

799. What is the magnification factor if an object measures 4 cm but the radiographic image is 8 cm?

A. 2X
B. 3X
C. 4X
D. 6X

A

800. Which of the following will occur when the tube angle is decreased?

A. The image will be foreshortened
B. Contrast will be lower
C. Shape distortion will decrease
D. Size distortion will increase

C

801. Which of the following will occur when the OID is decreased?

A. The image will be magnified
B. The image will be minified
C. The image is closer to actual size
D. The image will be elongated

C

802. Which of the following will have the greatest effect on size distortion?

A. SID
B. OID
C. Focal spot size
D. Image size

B

803. What advantage is there to magnifying an object?

1. Recorded detail increases
2. Small objects become visible
3. There is less distortion

A. 1 only
B. 2 only
C. 1 & 2 only
D. 1, 2 & 3

B

804. An x-ray tube that is designed for magnification radiography is referred to as what?

A. A fractional-focus tube
B. A mini-tube
C. A macro-tube
D. A radiographic enlarger

A

805. If the SID is increased the same as the OID, what will the resultant radiograph show?

A. No change in size distortion
B. An increase in size distortion
C. A decrease in size distortion
D. An elongated image

B

806. Which of the following affects shape distortion?

A. SID
B. OID
C. Focal spot size
D. X-ray tube angulation

D

807. Changing the shape of an object is called what?

A. Magnification
B. Distortion
C. Minification
D. Definition

B

808. To avoid shape distortion, which of the following must be paid close attention to?

A. SID
B. Part angulation
C. Part-to-table top distance
D. SOD

B

809. Which of the following can be done to help compensate for an angled part?

A. Angle the tube in the opposite direction
B. Angle the image receptor in the opposite direction
C. Align the tube, part and image receptor
D. Have the patient bend over

C

810. How does magnification affect the radiographic quality?

1. Decreases recorded detail
2. Decreases density
3. Lowers contrast

A. 1 only
B. 2 only
C. 2 & 3 only
D. 1, 2 & 3

A

811. Size distortion is affected by which of the following?

A. Intrinsic factors
B. Geometric factors
C. Motion factors
D. Technical factors

B

812. Which of the following will produce the largest image?

A. 40" SID, 3" OID
B. 40" SID, 5" OID
C. 72" SID, 3" OID
D. 72" SID, 5" OID

B

813. If the central ray is perpendicular to the image receptor, but the part is angled, what will be the result?

A. Foreshortening
B. Elongation
C. Minification
D. Loss of density

A

DENSITY

814. Changing the mA controls which of the following?

A. Penetrating power of the x-ray beam
B. Quality of the x-ray beam
C. Quantity of the x-ray beam
D. Average photon energy of the x-ray beam

C

815. Which of the following represents the useful range of radiographic densities?

A. .10 to 1.0
B. .20 to 2.0
C. .25 to 2.5
D. .35 to 3.5

C

816. Which of the following describes a radiograph that is lacking radiographic density?

A. Overexposed
B. Underexposed
C. Overpenetrated
D. Underpenetrated

B

817. How much must the mAs be increased before a noticeable change in density can be seen?

A. 10%
B. 30%
C. 50%
D. 75%

B

818. Which of the following factors affects radiographic density?

1. SID
2. OID
3. Focal spot size

A. 1 only
B. 2 only
C. 1 & 3 only
D. 1, 2 & 3

A

819. Which of the following defines radiographic density?

A. Differences between blacks and whites
B. Overall blackness of the radiograph
C. Sharpness of the radiograph
D. Visibility of the detail

B

820. Which of the following factors does NOT affect radiographic density?

A. Screen speed
B. Grid ratio
C. Processing
D. Film-screen contact

D

821. Even though it is considered a primary factor, why should kVp NOT be used to control density?

A. Contrast will also change
B. Detail will also change
C. It will cause motion
D. The tube will overload

A

822. Which of the following factors affect radiographic density?

1. kVp
2. Heel effect
3. Radiographic film

A. 1 only
B. 1 & 2 only
C. 2 & 3 only
D. 1, 2 & 3

D

823. A graphic representation of the relationship between density and exposure is called what?

1. D log E curve
2. H & D curve
3. Characteristic curve

A. 1 & 2 only
B. 1 & 3 only
C. 2 & 3 only
D. 1, 2 & 3

D

824. The quantity of x rays produced is dependent upon which of the following?

A. mAs
B. SID
C. OID
D. SOD

A

825. Which of the following statements concerning fog density is true?

A. The age of the film causes fog
B. Overdevelopment causes fog
C. Darkroom safelights cause fog
D. Every film has the same base fog

B

826. Which of the following is considered the main factor in the control of radiographic density?

A. mAs
B. kVp
C. SID
D. OID

A

827. Which of the following factors have the greatest effect on radiographic density?

A. Focal spot sizes
B. Grid ratios
C. mAs
D. kVp

D

828. Fog will have the greatest adverse effect on which of the following?

A. Low density areas of the image
B. Middle range density areas of the image
C. High density areas of the image
D. Maximum density areas of the image

A

829. Which of the following will NOT contribute to the underexposure of a radiograph?

A. mA set too low
B. kVp set too low
C. SID set too high
D. Focal spot size too large

D

830. If the mA is increased, how must the time be changed in order to maintain the same density?

A. Increased
B. Decreased
C. Doubled
D. Reduced by one half

B

831. What is the primary function of the mAs as it relates to radiographic quality?

A. Control contrast
B. Control recorded detail
C. Control density
D. Control distortion

C

832. What determines the density of a radiograph?

A. The number of silver halide crystals reduced by developer
B. The number of silver halide crystals removed by fixer
C. The brightness of the viewboxes
D. The perception of the radiologist

A

833. Even though it is considered a primary factor, why should the SID NOT be used to control density?

A. Contrast will also change
B. Recorded detail will also change
C. It will cause motion
D. The tube will overload

B

834. Quantum mottle is the result of an insufficient number of x rays. What contributes to quantum mottle?

1. High mAs and low kVp techniques
2. High speed screens
3. High ratio grids

A. 1 only
B. 2 only
C. 3 only
D. 1 & 2 only

B

835. If a radiograph transmits 1/1000 of the incident light, what is its density?

A. 1.0
B. 2.0
C. 2.5
D. 3.0

D

836. The light emitted from a screen contributes to what percentage of the overall film density?

A. 25%
B. 55%
C. 85%
D. 95%

D

837. How are mA and seconds related to each other when used to maintain density?

A. Directly proportional
B. Inversely proportional
C. Mutually exclusive
D. No relationship exists

B

838. Which of these is the best method to reduce scatter radiation which causes fog, an unwanted density?

A. Collimation
B. Filtration
C. Compression
D. High speed screens

A

839. Why is automatic exposure control (AEC) useful in controlling radiographic density?

1. Density must remain constant
2. Faulty density causes repeats
3. Density greatly affects quality

A. 1 only
B. 1 & 3 only
C. 2 & 3 only
D. 1, 2 & 3

D

840. Which of the following may be the cause of an overexposed radiograph?

A. Developer temperature too low
B. OID too high
C. SID too low
D. Grid ratio too high

C

841. When using a single phase unit, if the kVp is increased 15%, how much must the mAs be reduced in order to maintain the same density?

A. 15%
B. 25%
C. 50%
D. 100%

C

842. Which of the following describes the blackness of a radiograph?

A. Speed
B. Density
C. Gamma
D. Fog

B

843. If the exposure time is cut in half, how must the mA be adjusted to maintain the same density?

A. Cut in half
B. Reduced 2 times
C. Doubled
D. Increased 4 times

C

844. The density of a film will depend on which of the following factors?

1. Speed of film
2. Latitude of film
3. Gamma of film

A. 1 only
B. 2 only
C. 1 & 3 only
D. 1, 2 & 3

A

845. How does the base of an x-ray film affect the density of the radiograph?

A. It does not effect the density
B. It reduces density because it is clear
C. It adds to the density
D. It adds to the fog density

C

846. Which of the following film characteristics can be determined from an H and D curve?

1. Speed
2. Contrast
3. Base plus fog

A. 1 & 2 only
B. 1 & 3 only
C. 2 & 3 only
D. 1, 2 & 3

D

847. Which of the following screen speeds will produce the greatest density on a radiograph?

A. 50
B. 100
C. 200
D. 400

D

848. Which of the following could cause excessive density on a radiograph?

1. Contaminated fixer
2. Exhausted developer
3. Dryer temperature too high

A. 1 only
B. 2 only
C. 3 only
D. 1 & 2 only

B

849. A light radiograph may be caused by which of the following?

1. Grid cut-off
2. SID too low
3. Grid ratio too low

A. 1 only
B. 2 only
C. 3 only
D. 1 & 3 only

A

CONTRAST

850. Which of the following scales of contrast will produce a more consistent radiographic quality?

A. Short scale
B. Long scale
C. Narrow scale
D. Low scale

B

851. Subject contrast relates to which of the following?

A. The patient
B. The materials
C. The kVp
D. The scale of contrast

A

852. An H & D curve that demonstrates a steep curve represents a film with which of the following?

A. Low fog
B. High speed
C. High contrast
D. Low density

C

853. How will the use of radiographic grids affect the contrast of a radiograph?

A. Produce higher contrast
B. Produce lower contrast
C. Eliminate contrast
D. Have no effect on contrast

A

854. Which of the following factors would be used to control contrast?

A. mAs
B. kVp
C. SID
D. OID

B

855. Which of the following is defined as the ability of a film to record a wide range of densities?

A. Film speed
B. Film contrast
C. Film gamma
D. Film latitude

D

856. When using iodinated contrast agents and three-phase equipment, the kVp should NOT exceed what?

A. 50 kVp
B. 60 kVp
C. 70 kVp
D. 80 kVp

C

857. Which of the following affect subject contrast?

1. Size of patient
2. Part being radiographed
3. Type of tissue

A. 1 & 2 only
B. 1 & 3 only
C. 2 & 3 only
D. 1, 2 & 3

D

858. Which of the following directly influences radiographic contrast?

A. mA
B. SID
C. Grid ratio
D. Exposure time

C

859. Low energy radiation will result in which of the following?

A. Short scale contrast
B. Medium scale contrast
C. Long scale contrast
D. Low scale contrast

A

860. How will high kVp techniques affect radiographic contrast?

A. Produce higher contrast
B. Produce lower contrast
C. Produce higher contrast in obese patients
D. Will have no effect on contrast

B

861. The quality of an x-ray beam is determined by which of the following?

A. mAs
B. kVp
C. SID
D. Focal spot size

B

862. The difference in density between adjacent areas is a definition for which of the following?

A. Density
B. Contrast
C. Distortion
D. Recorded detail

B

863. How will increasing screen speed affect radiographic quality?

A. Produce higher contrast
B. Produce greater latitude
C. Produce lower contrast
D. Produce less density

A

864. Which of the following grid ratios should be used to maintain contrast when using over 100 kVp?

A. 5:1
B. 6:1
C. 8:1
D. 12:1

D

865. Which of the following affects radiographic contrast?

1. Radiographic film
2. Developer temperature
3. Screen speed

A. 1 only
B. 1 & 3 only
C. 2 & 3 only
D. 1, 2 & 3

D

866. How would an image with just a few, wide density differences be described?

A. High density
B. Low distortion
C. High contrast
D. Low recorded detail

C

867. Which of the following techniques will produce a radiograph with the highest contrast?

A. 50 mAs, 50 kVp
B. 30 mAs, 60 kVp
C. 15 mAs, 70 kVp
D. 10 mAs, 80 kVp

A

868. Increasing kVp will result in which of the following?

A. Producing higher contrast
B. Increasing photon energy
C. Decreasing photon energy
D. Decreasing distortion

B

869. Which of the following describes a short scale of contrast?

A. High contrast
B. Low contrast
C. High number of density differences
D. Greater film latitude

A

870. Which of the following will have the greatest effect on radiographic contrast?

A. Tube filtration
B. Close collimation
C. Focal spot size
D. Eliminating scatter radiation

D

871. Why is contrast needed in a radiographic image?

1. Makes detail visible
2. Increases sharpness of detail
3. Decreases need for distortion

A. 1 only
B. 2 only
C. 3 only
D. 1 & 2 only

A

872. Which of the following will produce a longer scale of contrast?

A. Increasing screen speed
B. Increasing kVp
C. Increasing grid ratio
D. Increasing SID

B

873. Scatter radiation will have the greatest effect on which of these radiographic qualities?

A. Recorded detail
B. Density
C. Contrast
D. Distortion

C

874. Which of the following statements is true?

A. High kVp, high contrast
B. High kVp, low contrast
C. High kVp, short scale
D. High kVp, low density

B

875. Which of the following statements is true?

A. A long scale has few densities
B. A long scale is high contrast
C. A long scale of contrast is usually preferred
D. High contrast has a lot of densities

C

876. The number of density differences in a radiograph refers to which of the following?

A. Subject contrast
B. Object contrast
C. Intrinsic contrast
D. Scale of contrast

D

877. Which of the following will produce a lower contrast in a radiograph?

1. High kVp
2. Improper collimation
3. Outdated film

A. 1 only
B. 1 & 3 only
C. 2 & 3 only
D. 1, 2 & 3

D

878. Which of the following screen speeds would produce a radiograph with low contrast?

A. 50
B. 100
C. 200
D. 400

A

879. How does a small increase in developer temperature affect radiographic contrast?

A. Produces higher contrast
B. Produces lower contrast
C. Eliminates contrast
D. Has no effect on contrast

A

880. Why is direct exposure film NOT recommended for modern day radiography?

A. Too much contrast
B. Not enough contrast
C. Requires long exposure times
D. Increases patient exposure

D

881. Which of the following radiographic procedures requires a long scale of contrast?

A. Lumbar spine
B. Chest
C. Myelography
D. Angiography

B

882. As contrast lowers, how is the number of densities in the image affected?

A. Increases
B. Decreases
C. Remains the same
D. Varies from image to image

A

883. Which of the following factors will NOT have an effect on radiographic contrast?

A. Patient
B. Grid ratio
C. SID
D. Radiation fog

C

884. Which of the following factors will NOT have an effect on film contrast?

A. Base plus fog
B. Maximum density
C. Manufacturer
D. Type of procedure

D

885. Which of the following would NOT be used as contrast media in radiography?

A. Air
B. Saline
C. Barium sulfate
D. Sodium iodide

B

886. Which of the following may lower radiographic contrast on a film?

1. Outdated film
2. Faulty safelight filter
3. Contaminated developer

A. 2 only
B. 3 only
C. 1 & 3 only
D. 1, 2 & 3

D

887. Subject contrast will be the lowest with which of the following body types?

A. Sthenic
B. Asthenic
C. Hyposthenic
D. Hypersthenic

D

888. Which of the following determines the visibility of detail in a radiograph?

A. Density and distortion
B. Contrast and recorded detail
C. Density and contrast
D. Density, contrast and recorded detail

C

889. Which of the following accessories can be used to demonstrate a scale of contrast or test for contrast?

A. Densitometer
B. Penetrometer
C. Rate meter
D. Wire mesh

B

890. What are the advantages of using high kVp techniques?

1. Less patient exposure
2. Longer tube life
3. All parts are well penetrated

A. 1 only
B. 1 & 3 only
C. 2 & 3 only
D. 1, 2 & 3

D

891. How will an air gap technique affect radiographic contrast?

A. Produce higher contrast
B. Produce lower contrast
C. Eliminate contrast
D. Have no effect on contrast

A

892. Which of the following describes a long scale of contrast?

A. High contrast
B. Low contrast
C. Less film latitude
D. Low number of density differences

B

893. How will an increase in radiographic fog affect contrast?

A. Contrast will be higher
B. Contrast will be lower
C. Contrast will be eliminated
D. Contrast will remain the same

B

894. Contrast can be measured from an H & D curve by finding the slope of which of the following parts?

A. Toe
B. Shoulder
C. Threshold
D. Straight line portion

D

895. Film A, in this H & D curve, represents which of the following?

A. Lowest fog
B. Lowest speed
C. Highest contrast
D. Highest latitude

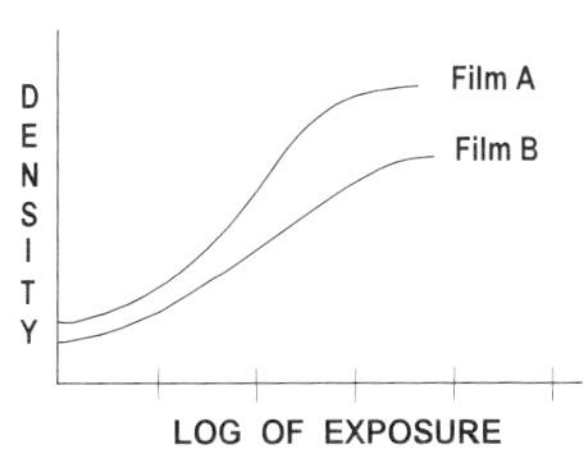

C

TECHNIQUE PROBLEMS

896. If using a three-phase generator, which of the following will have the greatest effect on increasing density?

A. 10% increase in kVp
B. 25% increase in SID
C. 50% increase in mAs
D. 75% increase in grid ratio

A

897. If the SID is halved, which of the following changes must be made in order to maintain the same density?

A. mAs halved
B. mAs reduced by 4X
C. mAs doubled
D. mAs increased 4X

B

898. If the mAs is 30 and the time is .1, the mA setting must be what?

A. 100 mA
B. 200 mA
C. 300 mA
D. 400 mA

C

899. How much mAs will be generated if the control panel is set at 200 mA and 1/5 second?

A. 20 mAs
B. 40 mAs
C. 80 mAs
D. 100 mAs

B

900. A single-phase technique of 300 mA, 1/10 second and 60 kVp is to be changed to 70 kVp, what would the new time be?

A. 1/40 second
B. 1/20 second
C. 1/3 second
D. 1/5 second

B

901. How much must the mAs be increased when changing from no grid to an 8:1 grid?

A. 2X
B. 3X
C. 4X
D. 5X

C

902. If the mA is set at 400 and the mAs obtained is 80, what must the time be set at?

A. .1 second
B. .2 second
C. .4 second
D. .8 second

B

903. In order to maintain density, if a technique of 200 mA, .2 second and 70 kVp is changed to .1 second, what is the new kVp?

A. 50 kVp
B. 60 kVp
C. 80 kVp
D. 90 kVp

C

904. How much must the mAs be decreased if a 200 speed screen is replaced by a 400 speed screen?

A. 25%
B. 50%
C. 3X
D. 4X

B

905. If 60 mAs is obtained and the time setting was .2 second, the mA must have been set at what?

A. 100 mA
B. 200 mA
C. 300 mA
D. 400 mA

C

906. A technique of 150 mA, 3/20 second and 100 kVp could be changed to 300 mA, _____ seconds and 85 kVp.

A. 3/20
B. 3/10
C. 1/15
D. 1/30

A

907. When going from a 16:1 grid to a 6:1 grid how must the mAs be adjusted?

A. Doubled
B. Reduced by 1/2
C. Tripled
D. Reduced by 1/3

B

908. For single-phase equipment, time can be decreased by 1/2 if the kVp is increased by what percentage?

A. 10%
B. 15%
C. 25%
D. 50%

B

909. At 60 kVp (single-phase), how much must the kVp be increased in order to double the density of the radiograph?

A. 6 kVp
B. 7 kVp
C. 8 kVp
D. 9 kVp

D

910. Which of the following mA and time settings will produce the greatest radiographic density?

A. 100 mA, 1/2 second
B. 200 mA, 1/4 second
C. 300 mA, 1/5 second
D. 400 mA, 1/8 second

C

911. If 50 mAs provides an optimum density at 40", how much mAs is necessary at 80"?

A. 12 mAs
B. 25 mAs
C. 100 mAs
D. 200 mAs

D

912. How many milliseconds are in .05 seconds?

A. 5
B. 50
C. 500
D. 5000

B

913. How much should kVp be increased for each additional centimeter of tissue to be penetrated?

A. 1 kVp
B. 2 kVp
C. 3 kVp
D. 4 kVp

B

914. How much should kVp be increased when radiographing a part in an orthopedic cast?

A. 5 kVp
B. 10 kVp
C. 15 kVp
D. 25 kVp

B

915. An exposure with a 12:1 grid requires 40 mAs, how much mAs should be used if no grid was used?

A. 2 mAs
B. 4 mAs
C. 8 mAs
D. 16 mAs

C

916. If an exposure time of 1/20 second was used, how many dots should a spinning top test reveal?

A. 3
B. 6
C. 9
D. 12

B

917. If 40 mAs and 80 kVp were used with single-phase equipment, what should be used for three-phase equipment?

A. 40 mAs and 60 kVp
B. 40 mAs and 80 kVp
C. 80 mAs and 60 kVp
D. 80 mAs and 80 kVp

A

918. Which of the following techniques will result in the least radiation exposure to the patient?

A. 50 mAs, 80 kVp
B. 100 mAs, 70 kVp
C. 200 mAs, 60 kVp
D. All will produce the same exposure

A

919. Which of the following tomographic angles will produce the thinnest body section?

A. 10 degrees
B. 20 degrees
C. 30 degrees
D. 40 degrees

D

920. In the 60-80 kVp range, a 10 kVp increase will increase density how much?

A. 10%
B. 25%
C. 50%
D. 100%

D

921. How many centimeters are in 40"?

A. 80.9 cm
B. 100.0 cm
C. 101.6 cm
D. 160.0 cm

C

922. If motion is a problem, and 50 mAs is needed, which of the following mA stations should be selected?

A. 100 mA
B. 200 mA
C. 400 mA
D. 800 mA

D

923. How many heat units would be produced for a single-phase technique of 200 mA, .5 seconds and 60 kVp?

A. 100 H.U.
B. 1000 H.U.
C. 3000 H.U.
D. 6000 H.U.

D

924. Which of the following techniques will produce 40 mAs?

1. 100 mA, .4 second
2. 200 mA, .2 second
3. 400 mA, .1 second

A. 1 only
B. 1 & 2 only
C. 1 & 3 only
D. 1, 2 & 3

D

925. How can the fraction 1/5 be written in decimal form?

A. .10
B. .20
C. .25
D. .50

B

926. Which of the following metric cassette sizes is equivalent to a 10 x 12 inch cassette?

A. 18 x 24
B. 24 x 30
C. 30 x 35
D. 35 x 43

B

927. A technique of 200 mA, .5 second and 68 kVp can be changed to 400 mA, _____ second and 68 kVp.

A. .10
B. .15
C. .25
D. .50

C

928. If 60 mAs provides optimum density with 100 speed screens, how much mAs is needed with 200 speed screens?

A. 20 mAs
B. 30 mAs
C. 120 mAs
D. 200 mAs

B

929. Which of these sets of technical factors will produce an image with the longest scale of contrast?

A. 50 mA, 1.0 second, 70 kVp
B. 100 mA, .50 second, 80 kVp
C. 200 mA, .25 second, 90 kVp
D. All are equal

C

930. What is the formula for determining heat units for a three-phase, six pulse generator?

A. mA x time x kVp
B. mA x time x kVp x 1.35
C. mA x time x kVp x 1.41
D. 2(mA x time x kVp)

B

931. 100 mA at 3/5 second produces an optimum density. What would the mA be if the time is reduced to 1/5 second?

A. 200 mA
B. 300 mA
C. 400 mA
D. 500 mA

B

932. If 80 mAs is needed without screens, how much mAs is needed with screens with an intensification factor of 40?

A. 2 mAs
B. 4 mAs
C. 20 mAs
D. 40 mAs

A

933. For three-phase equipment, time can be decreased by 1/2 if the kVp is increased by what percentage?

A. 10%
B. 15%
C. 25%
D. 50%

A

934. Which of the following techniques will produce the greatest radiographic density?

A. 100 mA, .50 second, 80 kVp
B. 200 mA, .50 second, 70 kVp
C. 300 mA, .33 second, 80 kVp
D. 400 mA, .25 second, 70 kVp

C

935. Which of the following techniques will produce the greatest radiographic density?

A. 50 mAs, 70 kVp, 40"
B. 100 mAs, 70 kVp, 40"
C. 100 mAs, 70 kVp, 80"
D. 100 mAs, 80 kVp, 80"

B

936. Which of the following techniques will produce the greatest radiographic density?

A. 100 mAs, 60 kVp, 100 speed screens
B. 100 mAs, 60 kVp, 200 speed screens
C. 100 mAs, 70 kVp, 100 speed screens
D. 100 mAs, 70 kVp, 200 speed screens

D

937. Which of the following techniques will produce the highest contrast?

A. 50 mAs, 80 kVp, 5:1 grid
B. 100 mAs, 70 kVp, 8:1 grid
C. 100 mAs, 80 kVp, 8:1 grid
D. 200 mAs, 70 kVp, 5:1 grid

B

CHAPTER FOUR

RADIOGRAPHIC PROCEDURES

- Positioning Terminology (26 questions)
- Upper Extremities (74 questions)
- Lower Extremities (62 questions)
- Abdomen and Thorax (76 questions)
- Vertebral Column and Pelvis (64 questions)
- Abdominal Viscera (70 questions)
- Skull and Facial Bones (82 questions)

POSITIONING TERMINOLOGY

938. Standing erect, facing forward with the palms of the hands forward, describes which of the following?

A. Oblique position
B. Trendelenburg position
C. Anatomical position
D. Upright position

C

939. What is the name of the plane that divides the body into right and left halves?

A. Coronal plane
B. Sagittal plane
C. Midsagittal plane
D. Transverse plane

C

940. What is another name for the midsagittal plane?

A. Median plane
B. Middle plane
C. Mean plane
D. Coronal plane

A

941. What is the name of the plane that divides the body into anterior and posterior halves?

A. Transverse plane
B. Horizontal plane
C. Sagittal plane
D. Midcoronal or midaxillary plane

D

942. What is the name of a plane that lies at a right angle to the midsagittal plane?

A. Oblique plane
B. Vertical plane
C. Transverse plane
D. Sagittal plane

C

943. When a patient is lying on his back, he is said to be in which position?

A. Proximal
B. Lateral
C. Supine
D. Median

C

944. Which of the following terms refers to the direction the x-ray beam travels?

A. Position
B. Projection
C. View
D. Decubitus

B

945. What term is used to describe the front half of the body, a structure or an organ?

A. Superior
B. Palmar
C. Anterior
D. Dorsal

C

946. The term caudad or caudal refers to which of the following?

A. Towards the tail end or feet
B. Towards the head end
C. Towards the ventral surface
D. Towards the apex

A

947. What would the position be referred to if the patient was lying down and the x-ray tube was directed horizontally?

A. Recumbent
B. Trendelenburg
C. Decubitus
D. Supine

C

948. The body part _____ the image receptor is referenced when describing the term "position".

A. Farthest from
B. Nearest
C. Above
D. Behind

B

949. What term is used to describe a part of a structure that is nearest to the origin or source?

A. Proximal
B. Medial
C. Cephalic
D. Distal

A

950. What term is used to describe the back half of the body, a structure or an organ?

A. Inferior
B. Plantar
C. Posterior
D. Ventral

C

951. Which of the following terms describes a lateral movement away from the median plane of the body?

A. Abduction
B. Adduction
C. Circumduction
D. Flexion

A

952. A position in which the midsagittal plane does NOT form a right angle with the image receptor or CR, is said to be a/an _____.

A. AP
B. PA
C. Lateral
D. Oblique

D

953. The part of a structure or organ which lies nearest to the midline of the body is said to be what?

A. Distal
B. Proximal
C. Medial
D. Lateral

C

954. When a patient is lying on his abdomen, he is said to be in which position?

A. Proximal
B. Lateral
C. Prone
D. Supine

C

955. Which of the following terms describes angling the x-ray tube toward the head?

A. Cephalic
B. Caudal
C. Inferior
D. Trendelenburg

A

956. What term is used to describe a part of a structure that is farthest from the origin or source?

A. Proximal
B. Medial
C. Cephalic
D. Distal

D

957. Which positioning term refers to the side of or a side view?

A. Dorsal
B. Lateral
C. Distal
D. Proximal

B

958. Which of the following terms describes a movement toward the median plane of the body?

A. Extension
B. Flexion
C. Abduction
D. Adduction

D

959. Which term refers to the lower part, or that part farther away from the head end of the body?

A. Internal
B. Intrinsic
C. Inferior
D. Superior

C

960. To place the hand with the palm up describes which of the following movements?

A. Rotate
B. Pronate
C. Supinate
D. Circumduct

C

961. To turn in or inward describes which of the following movements?

A. Flex
B. Extend
C. Adduct
D. Invert

D

962. Which of the following terms refers to the sole of the foot?

A. Plantar
B. Visceral
C. Parietal
D. Extrinsic

A

963. To straighten or stretch out the arm would be to _____ the elbow.

A. Flex
B. Extend
C. Rotate
D. Pronate

B

UPPER EXTREMITIES

964. How many carpal bones are there in a normal right wrist?

A. 2
B. 4
C. 6
D. 8

D

965. Which of the following bones is the longest?

A. 1st metacarpal
B. 2nd metacarpal
C. Ulna
D. Radius

C

966. What are the names for the bones located in the palm of the hand?

A. Phalanges
B. Metacarpals
C. Tarsals
D. Volars

B

967. What separates the head of the humerus from the shaft of the humerus?

A. Anatomical neck
B. Intertubercular groove
C. Lesser tubercle
D. Trochlea

A

968. The first metacarpal is located on which side of the hand?

A. Lateral
B. Medial
C. Ulnar
D. Inside

A

969. Why is this oblique radiograph of the hand NOT acceptable?

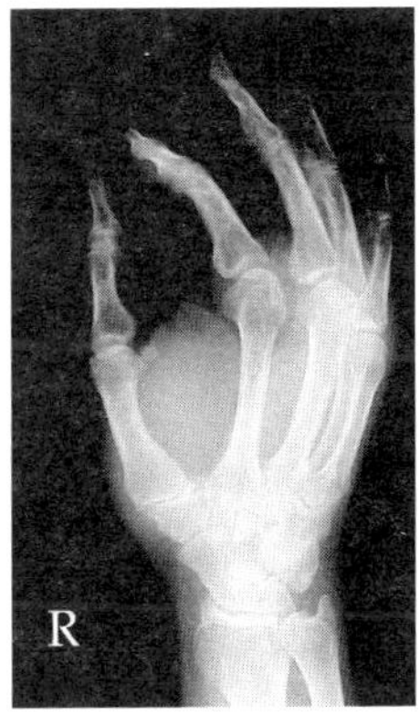

A. 1st digit is rotated
B. Metacarpals are superimposed
C. 5th distal phalanx is not visible
D. Soft tissue is visible

B

970. What are the joints called that are between the metacarpals and the proximal phalanges?

A. Interphalangeal joints
B. Carpometacarpal joints
C. Metacarpophalangeal joints
D. Synarthrodial joints

C

971. Which of the following articulates with the clavicle?

A. Scapula and humerus
B. Scapula and sternum
C. Humerus and sternum
D. Sternum and spine

B

972. Which carpal bone is most commonly fractured?

A. Scaphoid
B. Lunate
C. Hamate
D. Pisiform

A

973. The scapula is classified as what type of bone?

A. Long bone
B. Short bone
C. Irregular bone
D. Flat bone

D

974. Which of the following bones is in the proximal row of carpals?

A. Trapezoid
B. Triquetrum
C. Capitate
D. Hamate

B

975. Which of the following is NOT well demonstrated on an AP projection of the elbow?

A. Radial head
B. Radial tuberosity
C. Condyles of the humerus
D. Olecranon process

D

976. The trapezium articulates with which of the following?

A. Hamate
B. Pisiform
C. 1st metacarpal
D. 5th metacarpal

C

977. Which bones make up the elbow joint?

A. Radius and ulna
B. Radius and humerus
C. Radius, ulna and humerus
D. Capitulum, trochlea and radial head

C

978. Which of the following is the largest bone in the upper extremity?

A. Radius
B. Ulna
C. Humerus
D. Clavicle

C

979. The actual wrist joint is made up of which two bones?

A. Scaphoid and lunate
B. Ulna and pisiform
C. Ulna and scaphoid
D. Radius and scaphoid

D

980. The acromion is located on which of the following bones?

A. Radius
B. Ulna
C. Clavicle
D. Scapula

D

981. Pronating the hand flat will put the thumb in what position?

A. AP
B. PA
C. Oblique
D. Lateral

C

982. Which of the following positions will best demonstrate the scaphoid bone in the wrist?

A. Ulnar flexion
B. Ulnar deviation
C. Lateral
D. Carpal canal

B

983. Which of the following is used to determine if there is any separation of the AC joint?

A. Patient erect, steep oblique
B. Patient erect, holding weights
C. Patient supine
D. 15^0 cephalic angle

B

984. Which carpal bone lies between the scaphoid and the triquetrum?

A. Lunate
B. Hamate
C. Capitate
D. Pisiform

A

985. Where does the central ray enter for an AP projection of the 1st digit (thumb)?

A. 1st metacarpophalangeal joint
B. 1st proximal interphalangeal joint
C. 1st distal interphalangeal joint
D. 1st carpophalangeal joint

A

986. Where does the central ray enter for a PA projection of the 3rd digit?

A. 3rd metacarpophalangeal joint
B. 3rd proximal interphalangeal joint
C. 3rd distal interphalangeal joint
D. 3rd carpophalangeal joint

B

987. Which of the following is necessary for a true lateral position of the elbow?

1. Hand placed in a lateral position
2. Elbow flexed 90^0
3. Humeral epicondyles superimposed

A. 1 & 2 only
B. 1 & 3 only
C. 2 & 3 only
D. 1, 2 & 3

D

988. A lateral position of the scapula requires which of the following?

A. Unaffected arm raised
B. Patient breathes shallowly
C. Spine of scapula parallel to the image receptor
D. Central ray to medial border

D

989. When radiographing the 2nd digit in the lateral position, which part of the digit is closest to the image receptor?

A. Palmar
B. Dorsal
C. Medial
D. Lateral

D

990. Where does the central ray enter for a PA projection of the hand?

A. 3rd carpometacarpal joint
B. 3rd metacarpophalangeal joint
C. 3rd interphalangeal joint
D. 3rd proximal carpal joint

B

991. What angle joins the medial and lateral border of the scapula?

A. Superior angle
B. Inferior angle
C. Lateral angle
D. Medial angle

B

992. What are the routine positions/projections for a wrist?

A. AP and lateral
B. PA and oblique
C. PA, oblique and lateral
D. PA, oblique and ulnar flexion

C

993. For a routine, lateral position of the wrist, which surface is nearest the image receptor?

A. Medial
B. Lateral
C. Posterior
D. Ventral

A

994. Which bone in the forearm is located laterally?

A. Radius
B. Ulna
C. Humerus
D. Scaphoid

A

995. Where does the trochlea lie in comparison to the capitulum?

A. Superior
B. Inferior
C. Medial
D. Lateral

C

996. At which end of the ulna is the styloid process located?

A. Medial
B. Lateral
C. Proximal
D. Distal

D

997. How many bones are in a normal, adult skeleton?

A. 100
B. 106
C. 200
D. 206

D

998. What is another name for the lateral border of the scapula?

A. Superior
B. Inferior
C. Axillary
D. Medial

C

999. Where is the scapular notch located?

A. Superior to the scapular spine
B. Inferior to the scapular spine
C. Inferior to the supraspinous fossa
D. Lateral to the acromion process

A

1000. Which of the following will place the humerus in a true lateral position?

A. Internal rotation
B. External rotation
C. Abduction
D. Adduction

A

1001. The capitullum of the humerus articulates with which of the following anatomical structures?

A. Styloid process of the radius
B. Head of the radius
C. Head of the ulna
D. Styloid process of the ulna

B

1002. To get the wrist nearest the image receptor for a PA projection, which of the following must be done?

A. Elbow flexed 90^0
B. Digits extended
C. Digits separated
D. Digits flexed

D

1003. The trochlea of the humerus articulates with which of the following anatomical structures?

A. Radial tuberosity
B. Head of the radius
C. Styloid process of the ulna
D. Trochlear notch of the ulna

D

1004. To prevent superimposition of the bones of the forearm, which of the following must be taken?

A. AP
B. PA
C. Oblique position
D. Lateral position

A

1005. Where is the anatomical neck of the humerus located in relation to the surgical neck?

A. Lateral
B. Superior
C. Inferior
D. Medial

B

1006. In this radiograph, what position is the elbow in?

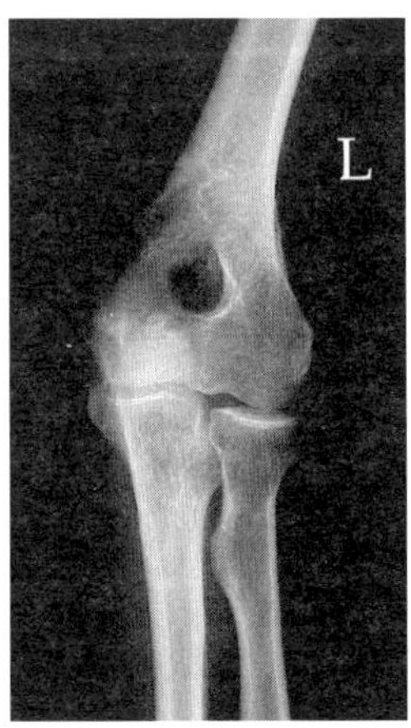

A. AP
B. 45^0 internal oblique
C. 45^0 external oblique
D. 90^0 lateral

C

1007. Which of the following anatomical structures would NOT be seen in a radiograph of the elbow?

A. Head of the radius
B. Olecranon process
C. Coronoid process
D. Styloid process of the radius

D

1008. Which two positions/projections are taken of a shoulder that has NOT been injured?

A. AP and external rotation
B. AP and PA
C. AP and transthoracic
D. AP internal and AP external rotation

D

1009. Which of the following positions/projections would best demonstrate the olecranon process of the ulna?

A. AP
B. 45^0 internal oblique
C. 45^0 external oblique
D. 90^0 lateral

D

1010. What is the name of the projection that can be palpated on the medial aspect of the humerus?

A. Olecranon process
B. Coronoid process
C. Coracoid process
D. Medial epicondyle

D

1011. Which of the following positions/projections would best demonstrate the coronoid process of the ulna?

A. AP
B. 45^0 internal oblique
C. 45^0 external oblique
D. 90^0 lateral

B

1012. The head of the humerus articulates with which part of the scapula?

A. Glenoid cavity
B. Olecranon fossa
C. Scapular notch
D. Styloid process

A

1013. The accuracy of a lateral elbow can be determined by the superimposition of which of the following?

A. Humeral condyles
B. Radius and ulna
C. Trochlea and radial head
D. Coronoid process and radial head

A

1014. Which of the following positions will best demonstrate the greater tubercle of the humerus?

A. AP internal rotation
B. AP external rotation
C. Transthoracic lateral
D. Transaxillary

B

1015. Which of the following cannot be palpated?

A. Styloid process of the ulna
B. Olecranon process
C. Radial tuberosity
D. Humeral epicondyles

C

1016. What is the name of the groove between the lesser and greater tubercles of the humerus?

A. Trochlear
B. Humeral
C. Intertubercular
D. Surgical

C

1017. Which of the carpal bones is "pea-shaped"?

A. Capitate
B. Pisiform
C. Lunate
D. Hamate

B

1018. Which of the following is the most likely location for a fracture of the humerus?

A. Anatomical neck
B. Surgical neck
C. Medial condyle
D. Lateral condyle

B

1019. Which of the following positions is used to demonstrate foreign bodies in the hand?

A. Tunnel
B. Carpal
C. Ulnar flexion
D. Lateral in extension

D

1020. What is the correct term for the armpit?

A. Fossa
B. Glenoid
C. Axilla
D. Semi-lunar

C

1021. How must the patient's arm be positioned for a good AP projection of the scapula?

A. Adducted
B. Abducted
C. Internally rotated
D. Externally rotated

B

1022. Which of the following positions could be used if there is an obvious fracture of the upper humerus?

A. AP internal rotation
B. AP external rotation
C. Transaxillary
D. Transthoracic lateral

D

1023. What is the most proximal end of the ulna called?

A. Styloid process
B. Olecranon process
C. Deltoid tuberosity
D. Trochlea

B

1024. What is the name of the joint between the two bones of the shoulder girdle?

A. Acromioclavicular joint
B. Shoulder joint
C. Sternoclavicular joint
D. Scapular notch

A

1025. How many phalanges are in the thumb?

A. 1
B. 2
C. 3
D. 4

B

1026. For the best recorded detail, which of the following positions/projections of the clavicle should be used?

A. AP
B. PA
C. Lateral
D. Oblique

B

1027. How many degrees is the hand rotated for an oblique position?

A. 15^0
B. 30^0
C. 45^0
D. 60^0

C

1028. Which two bones make up the shoulder girdle?

A. Clavicle and humerus
B. Clavicle and scapula
C. Scapula and humerus
D. Scapula and sternum

B

1029. What anatomical structures are referred to as the "knuckles"?

A. Metacarpophalangeal joints
B. Carpometacarpal joints
C. Interphalangeal joints
D. Intercarpal joints

A

1030. Which of the following is NOT a border of the scapula?

A. Lateral
B. Inferior
C. Superior
D. Medial

B

1031. How many interphalangeal joints are in the third digit?

A. 1
B. 2
C. 3
D. 4

B

1032. What is the name of the structure that separates the two posterior fossae of the scapula?

A. Scapular notch
B. Acromion process
C. Spine of the scapula
D. Coracoid process

C

1033. The extremities, the shoulder girdles and the pelvis make up which of the following?

A. Bony skeleton
B. Axial skeleton
C. Appendicular skeleton
D. False skeleton

C

1034. What is the name of the process that extends anteriorly from the scapula?

A. Acromion process
B. Coronoid process
C. Glenoid process
D. Coracoid process

D

1035. Where should the central ray enter for an AP projection of the shoulder joint?

A. Acromion process
B. Scapular notch
C. Glenoid process
D. Coracoid process

D

1036. How many degrees should the tube be angled for an AP projection of the clavicle?

A. 15^0 caudal
B. 15^0 cephalic
C. 45^0 caudal
D. 45^0 cephalic

B

1037. In this shoulder radiograph, the humerus is in which of the following positions?

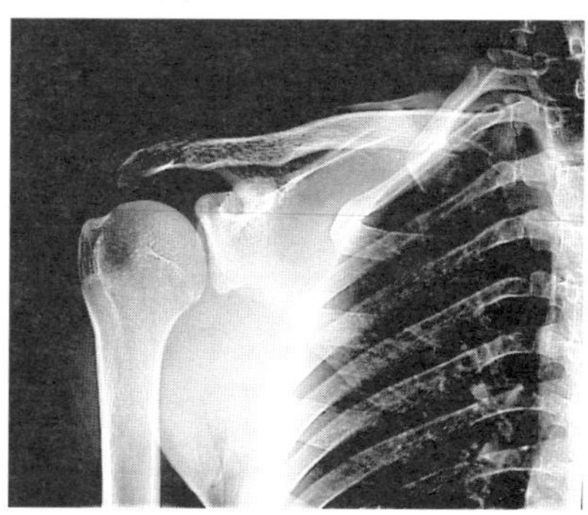

A. Lateral
B. AP internal rotation
C. AP external rotation
D. Transaxillary

C

LOWER EXTREMITIES

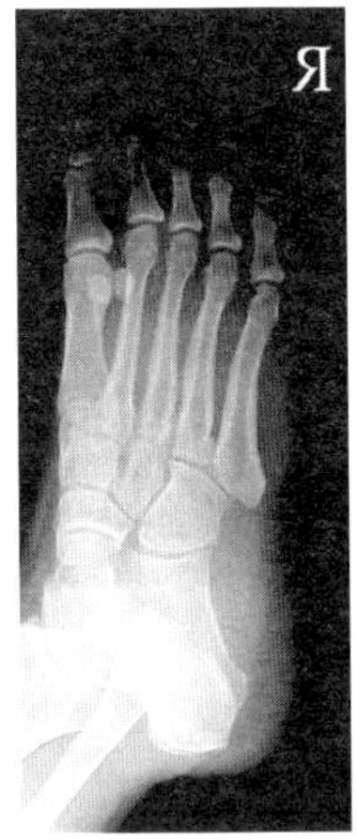

1038. Which of the following is NOT well demonstrated on this medial oblique projection of the foot?

A. Intertarsal joints
B. Intermetatarsal spaces
C. Tarsal bones
D. Ankle joint

D

1039. For this medial oblique projection of the foot, how many degrees should the foot be rotated?

A. 15^0
B. 30^0
C. 45^0
D. 60^0

B

1040. Where should the central ray enter for a dorsoplantar projection of the foot?

A. 3rd metatarsophalangeal joint
B. Base of the 3rd metatarsal
C. Anterior talus
D. Medial cuneiform

B

1041. What is the rounded process on the proximal, medial aspect of the femur called?

A. Medial epicondyle
B. Lesser tuberosity
C. Lesser trochanter
D. Femoral tuberosity

C

1042. When radiographing the hip in the AP projection, what should be done to the patient's foot?

A. Elevated
B. Rotated internally
C. Rotated externally
D. Abducted

B

1043. How many tarsal bones are there in the foot?

A. 3
B. 5
C. 7
D. 9

C

1044. The "frog" lateral is a common name given to a position for which of the following anatomical areas?

A. Intercondyloid fossa
B. Subtalar joint
C. Hip joint
D. Club foot

C

1045. What are the two small bones called that are located at the first metatarsophalangeal joint?

A. Sesamoids
B. Phalanges
C. Tarsals
D. Metatarsals

A

1046. For a cross-table lateral of the hip, where is the central ray directed?

A. Parallel to the shaft of the femur
B. Parallel to the neck of the femur
C. Perpendicular to the neck of the femur
D. Perpendicular to the acetabulum

C

1047. What is the most proximal end of the fibula called?

A. Head
B. Neck
C. Lateral malleolus
D. Apex

D

1048. When the patient is in a Cleaves position (frog), how are the patient's thighs positioned?

A. Adducted
B. Abducted
C. Elevated
D. Extended

B

1049. Which of the following tarsal bones articulates with the talus anteriorly?

A. Calcaneus (Os Calcis)
B. Cuboid
C. Cuneiform
D. Navicular

D

1050. Which of the following must be done for a properly positioned AP projection of the ankle?

1. Ankle joint flexed
2. Tube angled 10^0 cephalad
3. Plantar surface touching the image receptor

A. 1 only
B. 3 only
C. 2 & 3 only
D. 1, 2 & 3

A

1051. What is the area called that separates the medial and lateral femoral condyles posteriorly?

A. Intertrochanteric fossa
B. Olecranon fossa
C. Epicondyloid fossa
D. Intercondyloid fossa

D

1052. What is the radiographic examination of the menisci called?

A. Phlebography
B. Popliteal angiogram
C. Tibial radiography
D. Knee arthrography

D

1053. The medial malleolus, lateral malleolus and talus form which joint?

A. Knee
B. Ankle
C. Foot
D. Subtalar

B

1054. Where should the central ray be directed for an AP projection of the knee joint?

A. 1 cm proximal to the base of the patella
B. 1 cm distal to the apex of the patella
C. 1 cm distal to the base of the patella
D. Parallel to the patellar surface

B

1055. What view of the patella will be obtained with the patient prone and the affected knee flexed 90^0?

A. Settegast
B. Merchant
C. Hughston
D. Stecher

A

1056. Which of the following is necessary to demonstrate the intercondyloid fossa?

A. CR perpendicular to the knee joint
B. CR perpendicular to the lower leg
C. CR parallel to the patella
D. Knee fully flexed

B

1057. What is the most distal portion of the fibula called?

A. Apex
B. Lateral malleolus
C. Medial malleolus
D. Head

B

1058. For the frog-leg position of a unilateral hip, where is the central ray directed?

A. Perpendicular to the femoral neck
B. Parallel to the femoral neck
C. Parallel to the shaft
D. Perpendicular to the acetabulum

A

1059. What is the largest sesamoid bone in the body?

A. Calcaneus (Os Calcis)
B. Talus
C. Patella
D. Cuboid

C

1060. Which of the following is a common name for the position that demonstrates the intercondyloid fossa?

A. Shovel view
B. Sunrise view
C. Tunnel view
D. Skyline view

C

1061. Which direction and how many degrees must the x-ray tube be angled to best visualize the knee joint in an AP projection?

A. Cephalad, 5^0
B. Caudad, 5^0
C. Cephalad, 15^0
D. Caudad, 15^0

A

1062. What is the name of the largest bone in the lower leg?

A. Femur
B. Tibia
C. Fibula
D. Talus

B

1063. On which side of the foot does the cuboid lie?

A. Plantar
B. Dorsal
C. Medial
D. Lateral

D

1064. The term popliteal refers to which of the following anatomical areas?

A. Anterior knee
B. Posterior knee
C. Lateral knee
D. Medial knee

B

1065. What is the rounded process on the proximal, lateral aspect of the femur called?

A. Lateral epicondyle
B. Greater trochanter
C. Greater tuberosity
D. Femoral tuberosity

B

1066. The lateral cuneiform articulates with which of the following bones of the foot?

1. 3rd metatarsal
2. Cuboid
3. Navicular

A. 1 only
B. 1 & 2 only
C. 2 & 3 only
D. 1, 2 & 3

D

1067. What are the names of the bones that form the instep of the foot?

A. Tarsals
B. Phalanges
C. Metatarsals
D. Cuneiforms

C

1068. Which of the following terms relates to the top of the foot?

A. Plantar
B. Dorsal
C. Volar
D. Ventral

B

1069. What is the name of the bony projection on the tibial plateau?

A. Tibial tuberosity
B. Tibial tubercle
C. Intercondyloid eminence
D. Superior epicondyle

C

1070. What is the hollow portion of the shaft of a long bone called?

A. Osteum
B. Medullary cavity
C. Periosteum
D. Cortex

B

1071. Which of the following tarsal bones articulates with the talus inferiorly?

A. Calcaneus (Os Calcis)
B. Cuboid
C. Cuneiform
D. Navicular

A

1072. Which of the following serves to fasten muscles to bones?

A. Ligaments
B. Tendons
C. Extenders
D. Meniscus

B

1073. Which of the following positions/projections requires the foot vertical and the tube angled 40^0 cephalad?

A. AP ankle
B. Cross-table lateral hip
C. Plantodorsal, axial calcaneus
D. Dorsoplantar foot

C

1074. What is the name of the largest tarsal bone?

A. Talus
B. Cuboid
C. Calcaneus (Os Calcis)
D. Navicular

C

1075. What is the rounded projection on the anterior, proximal surface of the tibia called?

A. Tibial plateau
B. Tibial tuberosity
C. Intercondylar eminence
D. Tibial condyle

B

1076. Which side of the foot is closest to the image receptor for a lateral position of the foot?

A. Plantar
B. Dorsal
C. Lateral
D. Medial

C

1077. The medial cuneiform articulates with which of the following?

A. Cuboid
B. Calcaneus (Os Calcis)
C. First metatarsal
D. First phalanx

C

1078. Which of the following positions/projections will best show the space between the patella and the femur?

A. AP
B. Axial
C. Internal oblique
D. External oblique

B

1079. Which of the malleoli is part of the distal tibia?

A. Superior
B. Anterior
C. Medial
D. Lateral

C

1080. A medial oblique position of the foot will put which of the following structures closest to the image receptor?

A. Medial cuneiform
B. Cuboid
C. Talus
D. 5th metatarsal

A

1081. With the foot and lower leg rotated medially 45^0, what position of the ankle would be obtained?

A. AP
B. Semi-axial
C. Oblique
D. Steep lateral

C

1082. Which of the following bones articulates with the bases of the metatarsals?

A. Proximal phalanges
B. Distal phalanges
C. Tarsals
D. Tibia and fibula

C

1083. What is the name of the radiographic procedure where contrast medium is injected into the veins of the leg?

A. Lymphangiography
B. Arteriography
C. Scanography
D. Venography

D

1084. What is the term used to describe the inferior surface of the foot?

A. Dorsal
B. Plantar
C. Volar
D. Palmar

B

1085. How many phalanges are there in each foot?

A. 5
B. 7
C. 14
D. 24

C

1086. Where should the central ray enter for an AP projection of the 1st toe?

A. Interphalangeal joint
B. Proximal interphalangeal joint
C. Distal interphalangeal joint
D. Head of the 1st metatarsal

A

1087. Which anatomical landmarks are used to locate the neck of the femur?

A. Symphysis and greater trochanter
B. Symphysis and crest of the ilium
C. Symphysis and A.S.I.S.
D. Symphysis and ischial tuberosity

C

1088. Which of the following should NOT be seen in an AP radiograph of the hip if the femur is rotated correctly?

A. Lesser trochanter
B. Greater trochanter
C. Femoral neck
D. Intertrochanteric crest

A

1089. Which of the following would require a lateral rotation for its oblique position?

A. Hip
B. Knee
C. Ankle
D. 5th toe

D

1090. Which of the following positions/projections should be done if the patient has a suspected hip fracture?

A. AP and PA
B. AP and Cleaves
C. AP and cross-table lateral
D. Internal and external rotation

C

1091. Why does an AP projection of the foot require a 10^0 angle toward the calcaneus (os calcis)?

1. Toes have a natural 10^0 curvature
2. Intertarsal joints lie at a 10^0 angle
3. The strongest x rays go through the thickest part

A. 1 & 2 only
B. 1 & 3 only
C. 2 & 3 only
D. 1, 2 & 3

D

1092. Where should the central ray enter for a unilateral AP projection of the hip?

A. Acetabulum
B. Hip joint
C. Femoral neck
D. Mid-shaft of the femur

C

1093. What is the name of the concave, articular surface of the proximal tibia?

A. Intercondylar eminence
B. Tibial plateau
C. Tibial tuberosity
D. Anterior crest of the tibia

B

1094. Which of the following would be another name for the translateral hip projection?

1. Cross-table lateral
2. O.R. lateral
3. Inferosuperior projection

A. 1 & 2 only
B. 1 & 3 only
C. 2 & 3 only
D. 1, 2 & 3

D

1095. What is the best way to determine a true lateral position of the knee?

1. Femoral condyles superimposed
2. Malleoli on same transverse plane
3. Knee flexed 90^0

A. 1 only
B. 2 only
C. 1 & 3 only
D. 1, 2 & 3

A

1096. Where should the central ray enter for a medial oblique position of the 3rd toe?

A. 3rd metatarsophalangeal joint
B. 3rd distal interphalangeal joint
C. 3rd proximal interphalangeal joint
D. 3rd intertarsal joint

C

1097. What is another name for an AP projection of the foot?

A. Subtalar projection
B. Dorsoplantar projection
C. Plantodorsal projection
D. Semi-axial projection

B

1098. How many distal phalanges are there in a foot?

A. 4
B. 5
C. 12
D. 14

B

1099. What is the name of the largest bone in the lower extremity?

A. Fibula
B. Tibia
C. Femur
D. Calcaneus (Os Calcis)

C

ABDOMEN AND THORAX

1100. Which of the following structures serves as a common passageway for both food and air?

A. Trachea
B. Esophagus
C. Pharynx
D. Nasal cavity

C

1101. Which of the following positions/projections would best demonstrate the axillary portion of the right rib cage?

A. AP
B. RPO
C. RAO
D. Supine

B

1102. The thyroid cartilage of the larynx is at the level of which cervical vertebra?

A. 2
B. 4
C. 6
D. 8

B

1103. Which of the following is the preferred SID for radiography of the heart and lungs?

A. 36"
B. 40"
C. 60"
D. 72"

D

1104. Where is the trachea situated in relationship to the esophagus?

A. Lateral
B. Anterior
C. Posterior
D. Inferior

B

1105. What is the sac that encloses the lungs called?

A. Pleura
B. Pericardium
C. Mediastinum
D. Alveolar sac

A

1106. What is the area called where the bronchi enter the lungs?

A. Hilum
B. Pulmonary
C. Pleura
D. Alveoli

A

1107. Which of the following is NOT an artery that originates directly from the aortic arch?

A. Brachiocephalic artery
B. Right subclavian
C. Left carotid
D. Left coronary

B

1108. What is the portion of the lung that lies above the clavicles called?

A. Apex
B. Base
C. Costophrenic angle
D. Pleura

A

1109. What is the name of the valve that allows blood to pass from the left atrium to the left ventricle?

A. Mitral
B. Aortic
C. Tricuspid
D. Semilunar

A

1110. The right bronchus divides into ______ branches and the left bronchus into _____ branches.

A. 1, 2
B. 2, 1
C. 2, 3
D. 3, 2

D

1111. What is the name of the cartilage that prevents food from entering the larynx during swallowing?

A. Thymus
B. Thyroid
C. Epiglottis
D. Parathyroid

C

1112. Which of the following structures would NOT be found in the mediastinum?

A. Heart
B. Trachea
C. Esophagus
D. Epiglottis

D

1113. Which of the following are main branches of the trachea?

A. Alveoli
B. Laryni
C. Bronchioles
D. Bronchi

D

1114. Why are chest radiographs taken PA rather than AP?

A. To minimize heart magnification
B. So the patient can take in deeper breath
C. For better detail of the larynx
D. So patient cannot see you sweat

A

1115. What is the contracting phase of the heart called?

A. Dyspnea
B. Angina
C. Systole
D. Diastole

C

1116. What is the name for the small air sacs located at the distal ends of the bronchioles?

A. Pleura
B. Bronchi
C. Alveoli
D. Capillaries

C

1117. The xiphoid process is part of which of the following bones?

A. Scapula
B. Clavicle
C. Rib
D. Sternum

D

1118. What is the name of the area in the thoracic cavity located between the two lungs?

A. Intrathoracic space
B. Mediastinum
C. Interthoracic space
D. Cavitatum

B

1119. Which of the following positions would be used to show air-fluid levels on a patient who could NOT be done erect?

A. Prone
B. Trendelenburg
C. Sims
D. Lateral decubitus

D

1120. What breathing instructions should be given to a patient for a below the diaphragm radiograph of the ribs?

A. Inspiration
B. Expiration
C. Shallow breathing
D. Rapid breathing

B

1121. Which hemidiaphragm is usually located more superior?

A. Right
B. Left
C. Lateral
D. Medial

A

1122. What is the purpose of the thoracic duct?

A. Drains mediastinal fluid
B. Passes blood into the thorax
C. Conveys lymph into the left subclavian vein
D. Prevents blood from leaving thorax

C

1123. What is the lower, outer margin of the lung, at the junction of the ribs and diaphragm, called?

A. Base
B. Basilar angle
C. Costophrenic angle
D. Pleural junction

C

1124. Which of the following is NOT a part of the heart?

A. Superior vena cava
B. Left atrium
C. Right ventricle
D. Mitral valve

A

1125. Which gland is large when a person is young and almost disappears as an adult?

A. Pituitary
B. Adrenal
C. Thyroid
D. Thymus

D

1126. What is the main artery of the systemic circulation?

A. Brachiocephalic artery
B. Pulmonary artery
C. Aorta
D. Celiac trunk

C

1127. In which direction does the diaphragm move on inspiration?

A. Laterally
B. Inferiorly
C. Superiorly
D. Medially

B

1128. Why is the shortest possible exposure time necessary for chest radiography?

A. Patients cannot hold their breath
B. To eliminate heart motion
C. Less radiation to the patient
D. Improves radiographic contrast

B

1129. Why should the chin be extended when doing either a PA or a lateral chest radiograph?

A. To arch the patient's back
B. To demonstrate the lung apices
C. To assure the patient is erect
D. So the patient can breath deep

B

1130. Which of the following positions is used for a general scout radiograph of the abdomen?

A. Erect
B. Lateral decubitus
C. Dorsal decubitus
D. Supine

D

1131. Under what conditions should a chest be done supine rather than erect?

1. Patient is unconscious
2. Patient cannot sit up
3. Patient complains of dizziness

A. 1 & 2 only
B. 1 & 3 only
C. 2 & 3 only
D. 1, 2 & 3

D

1132. Which bone would be radiographed to demonstrate the manubrium?

A. Clavicle
B. Scapula
C. Sternum
D. Rib

C

1133. How many ribs should be showing above the diaphragm on a PA chest radiograph on deep inspiration?

A. 8
B. 10
C. 12
D. 14

B

1134. How many chambers are there in the heart?

A. 2
B. 3
C. 4
D. 6

C

1135. What are the basic positions/projections for a radiographic examination of the chest?

A. AP and left lateral
B. PA and right lateral
C. PA and left lateral
D. AP and right lateral

C

1136. Which of the following is the sac that surrounds the heart?

A. Pleura
B. Pericardium
C. Myocardium
D. Cardial membrane

B

1137. Why are the shoulders rotated forward when radiographing the chest in a PA projection?

1. To remove the scapulae from the lung fields
2. To get the chest closer to the image receptor
3. To allow a deeper inspiration

A. 1 only
B. 2 only
C. 1 & 3 only
D. 1, 2 & 3

A

1138. What are the first branches of the aorta that supply blood to the heart?

A. Coronary arteries
B. Brachiocephalic arteries
C. Subclavian arteries
D. Carotid arteries

A

1139. Which set of conditions would allow the diaphragm to descend to its most inferior position?

A. Patient supine, expiration
B. Patient supine, inspiration
C. Patient erect, expiration
D. Patient erect, inspiration

D

1140. Which of the following does NOT pass through the diaphragm?

A. Esophagus
B. Aorta
C. Trachea
D. Inferior vena cava

C

1141. The crest of the ilium is at the level of the vertebral interspace between lumbar vertebrae #_____ and #_____.

A. 1, 2
B. 2, 3
C. 3, 4
D. 4, 5

D

1142. In the fetus, the foramen ovale is located between which of the following chambers of the heart?

A. Right and left atrium
B. Right and left ventricle
C. Right atrium and ventricle
D. Left atrium and ventricle

A

1143. What is the name of the prominent, anterior end of thc iliac crcst?

A. Ischial tuberosity
B. Ischial spine
C. Anterior superior iliac spine
D. Anterior superior ischial spine

C

1144. Which of the following should be done to best visualize the sternum?

1. High kVp
2. Shallow, RAO
3. Short SID

A. 1 only
B. 2 only
C. 2 & 3 only
D. 1, 2 & 3

B

1145. What is the name of the large, thick muscle located on either side of the lumbar vertebrae?

A. Latissimus dorsi
B. Psoas
C. Deltoid
D. Columnar

B

1146. What are the blood vessels called that carry blood away from the heart?

A. Capillaries
B. Arteries
C. Veins
D. Venules

B

1147. What muscle separates the thoracic cavity from the abdominal cavity?

A. Psoas
B. Diaphragm
C. Lungular
D. Gluteal

B

1148. What are the breathing instructions for a patient having a routine chest radiograph?

A. Full expiration
B. Deep respiration
C. Deep inspiration
D. Shallow respiration

C

1149. What bony landmark is used for centering a supine abdominal radiograph?

A. Anterior superior iliac crest
B. Symphysis pubis
C. Iliac crest
D. 3rd lumbar vertebra

C

1150. What is the heart muscle called?

A. Myocardium
B. Pericardium
C. Circardium
D. Cardialum

A

1151. Which of the following structures should be seen on a good supine abdominal radiograph?

1. Lumbar transverse processes
2. Psoas muscles
3. Kidney outlines

A. 1 & 2 only
B. 1 & 3 only
C. 2 & 3 only
D. 1, 2 & 3

D

1152. How many pairs of ribs are there in a normal human skeleton?

A. 7
B. 12
C. 14
D. 24

B

1153. Which of the following reasons would NOT require an acute abdominal series?

A. A child swallowing a penny
B. Perforated hollow viscus
C. Intestinal obstruction
D. Abdominal infection

A

1154. What are the vessels called that carry blood to and from the lungs?

A. Coronary
B. Systematic
C. Hilar
D. Pulmonary

D

1155. Which decubitus abdomen position would be done if there was a question of free air within the abdomen?

A. Left lateral decubitus
B. Right lateral decubitus
C. Supine decubitus
D. Prone decubitus

A

1156. What is the organ of voice called?

A. Larynx
B. Pharynx
C. Thymus
D. Epiglottis

A

1157. An air-fluid level cannot be seen on which of the positions of a standard abdominal series?

A. Erect abdomen
B. Erect chest
C. Supine
D. Lateral decubitus

C

1158. The aorta arises from which chamber of the heart?

A. Right atrium
B. Left atrium
C. Right ventricle
D. Left ventricle

D

1159. What do the letters K.U.B. stand for?

A. Dr. Kub
B. Kidneys, ureter, bladder
C. Kidneys, umbilical, bowel
D. Kidneys, ureter, bowel

B

1160. Which of the following is a reliable method for checking for rotation on a PA chest radiograph?

A. Mediastinal shift
B. Compare size of lungs
C. Symmetry of sternoclavicular joints
D. Elevation of costophrenic angles

C

1161. Which body plane is centered to the midline of the table for a supine abdominal radiograph?

A. Midtransverse
B. Midlambdoidal
C. Midcoronal
D. Midsagittal

D

1162. What is the inferior end of the sternum called?

A. Body
B. Manubrium
C. Angle
D. Xiphoid process

D

1163. How long should a patient be upright before the erect radiograph of an acute abdomen series can be taken?

A. 1 minute
B. 3 minutes
C. 5 minutes
D. 7 minutes

C

1164. Which heart valves close when the ventricles of the heart contract?

A. Semilunar valves
B. Tricuspid and mitral valves
C. Tricuspid and semilunar valves
D. Pulmonary and aortic valves

B

1165. Which position has the patient standing erect and leaning backward to rest his/her shoulders against the image receptor?

A. Posterior oblique
B. Apical lordotic
C. Intrathoracic
D. Mediastinal tilt

B

1166. How many pairs of ribs are considered true ribs?

A. 3
B. 5
C. 7
D. 9

C

1167. How are the floating ribs best visualized?

A. Steep oblique
B. Lateral
C. Above the diaphragm
D. Below the diaphragm

D

1168. How many pairs of ribs are considered floating ribs?

A. 2
B. 3
C. 4
D. 5

A

1169. Where are the patient's arms placed for an erect lateral position of the chest?

A. On the hips
B. By the patient's side
C. Over the patient's head
D. Behind the back

C

1170. When radiographing the sternum, which oblique is preferred?

A. LAO
B. RAO
C. LPO
D. RPO

B

1171. Which of the following is NOT considered part of the bony thorax?

A. Sternum
B. Ribs
C. Thoracic spine
D. Lumbar spine

D

1172. Which one radiograph is the most important in a rib series involving recent trauma?

A. Erect chest
B. RAO
C. LPO
D. Below the diaphragm

A

1173. What term describes any abnormal accumulation of air in the pleural space?

A. Hemothorax
B. Pneumothorax
C. Pleurothorax
D. Dyspnea

B

1174. What are the breathing instructions for a lateral sternum?

A. Inspiration
B. Expiration
C. Shallow breathing
D. Rapid breathing

A

1175. A patient hurts in the left anterior part of the thorax. Which oblique would show this area best?

A. LAO
B. RAO
C. RPO
D. Lateral

B

VERTEBRAL COLUMN AND PELVIS

1176. Which of the following is the proper tube angle for an AP projection of the coccyx?

A. 10^0 cephalad
B. 10^0 caudad
C. 25^0 cephalad
D. 25^0 caudad

B

1177. What is the name of the most anterior portion of a thoracic vertebra?

A. Body
B. Lamina
C. Vertebral arch
D. Spinous process

A

1178. The acetabulum articulates with which of the following?

A. Inferior articulating process
B. Superior articulating process
C. Transverse process
D. Femoral head

D

1179. The brain and the spinal cord make up which part of the nervous system?

A. Sympathetic
B. Autonomic
C. Central
D. Peripheral

C

1180. How many cervical vertebrae are there?

A. 3
B. 5
C. 7
D. 12

C

1181. Which of the following contains the cerebrospinal fluid?

A. Dura mater
B. Pia mater
C. Arachnoid
D. Subarachnoid space

D

1182. The natural curve of the lumbar spine is classified as what type?

A. Concave
B. Convex
C. Spondylotic
D. Scoliotic

A

1183. Which vertebrae have demifacets for the articulation of ribs?

A. Cervical
B. Thoracic
C. Lumbar
D. Sacral

B

1184. What is another name for the first cervical vertebra?

A. Odontoid
B. Arch
C. Axis
D. Atlas

D

1185. Which position/projection is necessary to demonstrate the intervertebral foramina of the cervical spine?

A. AP
B. 45^0 oblique
C. 90^0 lateral
D. Odontoid

B

1186. How much must the body be rotated for an oblique position of the sacroiliac joints?

A. 15^0
B. 25^0
C. 45^0
D. 70^0

B

1187. The AP projection of the pelvis requires the lower extremities to be placed in which position?

A. Internally rotated
B. Externally rotated
C. Flexed
D. Adducted

A

1188. What is the name of the bony landmark on the anterior portion of the iliac crest?

A. Anterior trochanter
B. Anterior superior tuberosity
C. Anterior posterior iliac spine
D. Anterior superior iliac spine

D

1189. A long exposure time (breathing technique) is useful for which of the following positions/projections?

A. AP cervical spine
B. 70^0 oblique thoracic spine
C. Lateral thoracic spine
D. Open mouth

C

1190. Which of the following anatomical parts is NOT related to the others?

A. Symphysis pubis
B. Ischial spine
C. Iliac crest
D. Ileum

D

1191. What is the name of the large foramen in the innominate bone?

A. Foramen ovale
B. Foramen magnum
C. Obturator foramen
D. Pelvic foramen

C

1192. Which vertebra has no body?

A. First cervical
B. Second cervical
C. Seventh cervical
D. First thoracic

A

1193. What is the purpose of having the patient flex his knees for an AP projection of the lumbar spine?

A. Better visualization of disk spaces
B. Intervertebral foramen seen better
C. Eliminates spine distortion
D. More comfortable

A

1194. How much must the patient be obliqued in order to visualize the zygapophyseal joints of the thoracic spine?

A. 30^0
B. 45^0
C. 70^0
D. 90^0

C

1195. What is the name of the upper, curved border of the ilium called?

A. Ischial tuberosity
B. Iliac crest
C. Iliac spine
D. Anterior superior iliac spine

B

1196. What are the lateral projections on a typical vertebra called?

A. Spinous processes
B. Articular processes
C. Transverse processes
D. Pedicles

C

1197. What is another name for the second cervical vertebra?

A. Atlas
B. Axis
C. Dens
D. Posterior arch

B

1198. What is the name of the joint between the two pubic bones?

A. Acetabulum
B. Hip joint
C. Pelvic joint
D. Symphysis pubis

D

1199. What position was used to produce this AP dens radiograph?

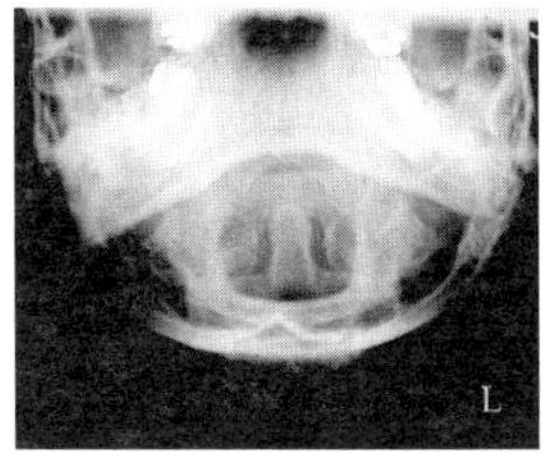

- A. Atlanto-axial
- B. Fuchs
- C. Haas
- D. Clements

B

1200. Where should the top of the image receptor be placed for an AP projection of the pelvis?

- A. Level of iliac crest
- B. Level of A.S.I.S.
- C. 2" above iliac crest
- D. Between iliac crest and symphysis

C

1201. How many movable joints can be visualized in an AP radiograph of a pelvis?

- A. 2
- B. 3
- C. 4
- D. 5

D

1202. How many thoracic vertebrae are there?

- A. 5
- B. 7
- C. 12
- D. 24

C

1203. Which of the following project off the posterior, lateral borders of the vertebral body?

- A. Pedicles
- B. Laminae
- C. Spinous process
- D. Articular processes

A

1204. Which of the following positions/projections will best demonstrate the L5-SI joint?

- A. AP
- B. PA
- C. Oblique
- D. Lateral

D

1205. What is the name of the process that projects downward from the base of the transverse process?

A. Pars interarticularis
B. Inferior articulating process
C. Spinous process
D. Lamina

B

1206. What is an abnormal lateral curvature of the spine called?

A. Lordosis
B. Kyphosis
C. Scoliosis
D. Meiosis

C

1207. Which of the following is NOT a part of a typical lumbar vertebra?

A. Body
B. Spinous process
C. Transverse foramen
D. Inferior articulating process

C

1208. Which of the following is true concerning the differences between a male and female pelvis?

A. Female pelvis is broader
B. Female pelvis is narrower
C. Female pubic arch is less angled
D. Female inlet is oval shaped

A

1209. How many lumbar vertebrae are there?

A. 5
B. 7
C. 12
D. 26

A

1210. What type of natural curve is found in the thoracic spine?

A. Concave
B. Convex
C. Scoliotic
D. Myoptic

B

1211. Rotation of the skull takes place between which of the following cervical vertebrae?

A. Cl and C2
B. C2 and C3
C. C4 and C5
D. C6 and C7

A

1212. What is the posterior, bony ring of a typical vertebra called?

A. Pedicle
B. Lamina
C. Vertebral body
D. Vertebral arch

D

1213. At what level is the image receptor centered for a lateral lumbosacral spine?

A. A.S.I.S.
B. Symphysis pubis
C. Iliac crest
D. First lumbar

C

1214. What is the most inferior portion of the pelvis called?

A. Ischial spine
B. Symphysis pubis
C. Ischial tuberosity
D. Inferior rami of the pubic bones

C

1215. How many degrees and in what direction should the tube be angled for an AP projection of the cervical spine?

A. 20^0 cephalad
B. 20^0 caudad
C. 30^0 cephalad
D. 30^0 caudad

A

1216. A 45^0 oblique of the lumbar spine is used to visualize which of the following?

A. Intervertebral spaces
B. Intervertebral foramina
C. Zygapophyseal joints
D. Bodies

C

1217. Which bone in the vertebral column is actually five separate vertebrae fused together?

A. Sternum
B. Sacrum
C. Coccyx
D. Innominate

B

1218. Which of the following projects posteriorly off the two laminae of a typical vertebra?

A. Transverse process
B. Superior articulating process
C. Inferior articulating process
D. Spinous process

D

1219. What is the technical name for the "Adam's apple"?

A. Pharynx
B. Larynx
C. Epiglottis
D. Thyroid cartilage

D

1220. What is the name of the process that projects upward from the body of the second cervical vertebra?

A. Spinous
B. Dens
C. Transverse
D. Superior

B

1221. Which of the following positions/projections would be required to demonstrate the mobility of the cervical spine?

A. Flexion and extension laterals
B. Inversion and eversion obliques
C. Internal and external rotation
D. AP and PA projections

A

1222. What is the name of the joint between the first and second cervical vertebrae?

A. Cervical joint
B. Cervical fusion
C. Atlantoaxial joint
D. Kyphotic joint

C

1223. What is the forward slipping of a vertebra called?

A. Cholelithiasis
B. Spondylolisthesis
C. Scoliosis
D. Slipped disk

B

1224. Which of the following passes through the transverse foramina of the cervical vertebrae?

A. Carotid artery
B. Jugular vein
C. Vertebral artery
D. Subclavian artery

C

1225. Which of the following angles is required for an AP projection of the sacrum?

A. 5^0 caudad
B. 5^0 cephalad
C. 15^0 caudad
D. 15^0 cephalad

D

1226. What is the name of the meningeal layer that is closest to the spinal cord?

A. Pia mater
B. Dura mater
C. Arachnoid
D. Subarachnoid

A

1227. Which of the following positions/projections is usually used to demonstrate the dens?

A. AP
B. AP open mouth
C. 45^0 oblique
D. Lateral

B

1228. Which of the following positions/projections would best demonstrate the transverse processes of the lumbar vertebrae?

A. AP
B. Lateral
C. 45^0 oblique
D. 70^0 oblique

A

1229. What is the name of the spongy pad that lies between the vertebrae?

A. Spinous disk
B. Intervertebral disk
C. Herniated disk
D. Intralumbar disk

B

1230. Which of the following positions/projections would best demonstrate the intervertebral spaces of the lumbar spine?

A. AP projection
B. Lateral
C. Mediolateral oblique
D. Lateromedial oblique

B

1231. What is the outer meningeal layer of the spinal cord called?

A. Dura mater
B. Pia mater
C. Arachnoid
D. Subarachnoid

A

1232. The spinal cord terminates at the level of which vertebra?

A. 12th thoracic
B. 2nd lumbar
C. 5th lumbar
D. 1st sacral

B

1233. Spina bifida is caused by which of the following?

A. Pedicles not fusing to the body
B. Pedicles not fusing with the laminae
C. Posterior laminae not fusing
D. Laminae and transverse processes fused

C

1234. What is the preferable SID for a lateral position of the cervical spine?

A. 36"
B. 40"
C. 60"
D. 72"

D

1235. What is the name of the opening through which the spinal cord passes?

A. Vertebral foramen
B. Intervertebral foramen
C. Transverse foramen
D. Obturator foramen

A

1236. The innominate bone is formed by the fusion of which three bones?

A. Pubis, trochanter, pelvis
B. Ilium, ischium, femur
C. Ileum, ischium, pubis
D. Ischium, pubis, ilium

D

1237. Which of the cervical vertebrae has the most prominent spinous process?

A. First
B. Third
C. Fifth
D. Seventh

D

1238. In the drawing of the typical vertebra below, the letter "B" represents which of the following anatomical parts?

A. Body
B. Lamina
C. Pedicle
D. Vertebral foramen

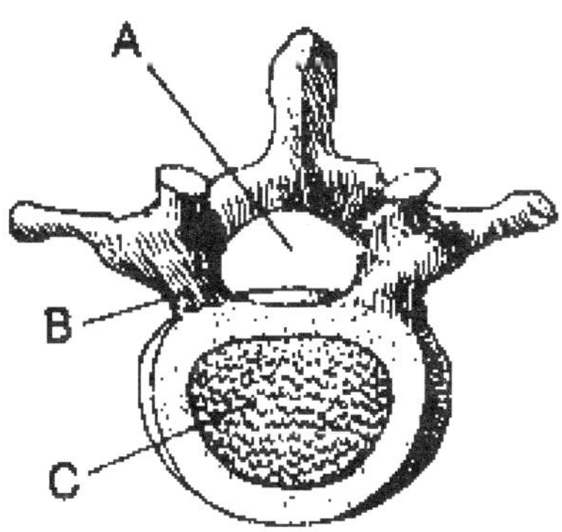

C

1239. How many pairs of spinal nerves are there?

A. 11
B. 21
C. 31
D. 41

C

ABDOMINAL VISCERA

1240. What is the name of the main bile duct that leads directly from the liver?

A. Common hepatic duct
B. Cystic duct
C. Common bile duct
D. Abdominal duct

A

1241. Which of the following describes the Valsalva maneuver?

A. Exhaling and holding breath out
B. Taking a deep breath and holding it
C. Bending over and touching ones toes
D. Taking a deep breath and straining down

D

1242. What is the proximal, pouch-like portion of the large intestine called?

A. Sigmoid
B. Cecum
C. Ileocecum
D. Ileum

B

1243. Which of the following conditions will produce the thinnest tomographic slice of the kidney?

A. 10^0 amplitude
B. 20^0 amplitude
C. 30^0 amplitude
D. 40^0 amplitude

D

1244. Patient preparation for an upper G.I. series would require which of the following?

A. High fat diet the evening before
B. Low fat diet the evening before
C. N.P.O. after midnight
D. Light breakfast the day of the procedure

C

1245. What is the name of the procedure that requires the injection of contrast media into the artery of the kidney?

A. Intravenous urography
B. Retrograde urography
C. Renal arteriography
D. Nephrotomography

C

1246. Which of the following is NOT part of the large intestine?

A. Right colic flexure
B. Jejunum
C. Ascending colon
D. Sigmoid

B

1247. What is the name of the air contrast study of the duodenum after the injection of an antispasmodic drug?

A. Air contrast G.I.
B. Air contrast duodenography
C. Hypotonic duodenography
D. Gastroscopy

C

1248. What is the meaning of deglutition?

A. The Chewing of food
B. The swallowing of food
C. The digestion of food
D. The elimination of food

B

1249. The portal system transports blood to which of the following organs?

A Spleen
B. Kidneys
C. Intestines
D. Liver

D

1250. At what level should the central ray enter for a RAO of the stomach of a sthenic patient?

A. T9
B. L2
C. L4
D. Iliac crest

B

1251. Which of the following organs would be located in the right upper quadrant of the abdomen?

A. Gall bladder
B. Spleen
C. Descending colon
D. Sigmoid

A

1252. What is the name of the opening in the proximal end of the stomach?

A. Sphincter of Oddi
B. Pyloric portion
C. Cardiac orifice
D. Hiatus

C

1253. Which of the following describes the term ileus?

A. Intestinal obstruction
B. Enlarged bowel
C. Distended stomach
D. Abdominal infection

A

1254. For an AP projection of the abdomen, the central ray is placed at the level of which anatomical structure?

A. Iliac crest
B. Symphysis pubis
C. Xiphoid process
D. A.S.I.S.

A

1255. A patient with a possible perforated ulcer would require which of the following procedures?

A. U.G.I. with thin barium
B. U.G.I. with thick barium
C. U.G.I with Gastrografin
D. U.G.I with air contrast

C

1256. What is the radiographic examination of the gall bladder called?

A. Biliography
B. Choleangiography
C. Cholecystography
D. Cystography

C

1257. What is the name of the organ that lies within the duodenal loop?

A. Spleen
B. Pancreas
C. Adrenal
D. Gall bladder

B

1258. The patient preparation for a barium enema would require which of the following?

A. Perfectly clean colon
B. Completely empty stomach
C. Totally sedated patient
D. N.P.O. two days prior to examination

A

1259. Which decubitus position is preferred for demonstrating air and fluid levels in the abdomen?

A. Dorsal decubitus
B. Ventral decubitus
C. Right lateral decubitus
D. Left lateral decubitus

D

1260. What is the name of the largest blood vessel in the abdomen?

A. Celiac
B. Renal
C. Aorta
D. Iliac

C

1261. Which of the following is supplied by the superior mesenteric artery?

A. Small intestine
B. Spleen
C. Liver
D. Pancreas

A

1262. When should the timing for a small bowel series begin?

A. When the patient enters the x-ray room
B. When the patient swallows the barium
C. When the radiologist completes fluoroscopy
D. Whenever the technologist wants

B

1263. Which of the following positions is routine for a small bowel radiograph?

A. Supine abdomen
B. Prone abdomen
C. Oblique abdomen
D. Erect abdomen

B

1264. The umbilicus lies at the level of which of the following?

A. 2nd and 3rd lumbar
B. 3rd and 4th lumbar
C. 4th and 5th lumbar
D. 5th lumbar and 1st sacral

B

1265. Which of the following abdominal organs produces and secretes digestive enzymes?

A. Gall bladder
B. Duodenum
C. Spleen
D. Pancreas

D

1266. Which of the following positions would the patient be in during the insertion of an enema tip?

A. Sims' position
B. Trendelenburg position
C. Fowler's position
D. Prone position

A

1267. What is the name of the S-shaped portion of the colon that lies proximal to the rectum?

A. Descending colon
B. Left colic flexure
C. Cecum
D. Sigmoid colon

D

1268. Which of the following positions will best demonstrate the pylorus and duodenal loop?

A. Supine
B. 45^0 LAO
C. 45^0 RAO
D. Prone

C

1269. An upper G.I. series on a hypersthenic patient would require what kind of an adjustment of the central ray?

A. 2" higher than normal
B. 2" lower than normal
C. More medial than normal
D. No adjustment would be needed

A

1270. Which of the following describes the blood vessels that supply the abdomen?

A. Pulmonary circulation
B. Lymphatic circulation
C. Appendicular circulation
D. Systemic circulation

D

1271. Which of the following positions will best demonstrate the left colic (splenic) flexure?

A. Supine
B. Prone
C. RAO
D. LAO

D

1272. What is the name of the most proximal portion of the stomach?

A. Pylorus
B. Greater curvature
C. Fundus
D. Body

C

1273. In tomography, the objective plane is at the same height as which of the following?

A. Fulcrum
B. Table top
C. Amplitude
D. SID

A

1274. In which of the following organs would Henle's loop be located?

A. Liver
B. Kidney
C. Adrenal
D. Pancreas

B

1275. Which of the following positions would best demonstrate the rectum filled with barium?

A. RPO
B. Supine
C. Lateral
D. Erect

C

1276. What is the name of the large muscles that lie along the lateral borders of the lumbar vertebrae?

A. Latissimus dorsi
B. Deltoid
C. Psoas
D. Intervertebral

C

1277. Which of the following organs have folds that are referred to as haustra?

A. Stomach
B. Large intestine
C. Gall bladder
D. Small intestine

B

1278. Which kidney is placed parallel to the image receptor when a 30^0 RPO radiograph is taken?

A. Right
B. Left
C. Both are parallel
D. Both are perpendicular

B

1279. The gall bladder will be located near the vertebrae in which of the following body types?

A. Asthenic
B. Sthenic
C. Hypersthenic
D. Average

A

1280. The majority of food digestion takes place in which of the following organs?

A. Stomach
B. Duodenum
C. Small intestine
D. Large intestine

B

1281. A double contrast enema consists of which of the following?

A. AP and PA abdominal radiographs
B. A second examination of the large intestine
C. A double volume large intestine examination
D. Air and barium exam of the large intestine

D

1282. The abdominal aorta bifurcates into right and left ___ arteries.

A. Mesenteric
B. Iliac
C. Renal
D. Femoral

B

1283. What is the name of the duct that transports bile from the gall bladder?

A. Hepatic duct
B. Cystic duct
C. Duodenal duct
D. Common hepatic duct

B

1284. What is the name of the examination where contrast media is injected into the uterus and uterine tubes?

A. Urography
B. Pelvimetry
C. Placentography
D. Hysterosalpingography

D

1285. What is the name of the tube that passes from the kidney to the urinary bladder?

A. Urinary duct
B. Urethra
C. Uterus
D. Ureter

D

1286. Which of the following would NOT be found in the urinary system?

A. Nephron
B. Glomerulus
C. Adrenal
D. Calyx

C

1287. Which of the following positions/projections would best demonstrate a hiatal hernia?

A. AP
B. Lateral
C. RAO
D. LAO

A

1288. In the hypersthenic patient, how does the stomach lie?

A. Low and vertical
B. Low and horizontal
C. High and vertical
D. High and horizontal

D

1289. In which of the abdominal regions will the duodenum be located?

A. Hypogastric
B. Epigastric
C. Umbilical
D. Left hypochondriac

C

1290. Which of the following is NOT an accessory organ of the digestive system?

A. Pancreas
B. Gall bladder
C. Liver
D. Spleen

D

1291. What is the name of the proximal, funnel shaped portion of the ureter called?

A. Calyx
B. Cortex
C. Renal pyramid
D. Renal pelvis

D

1292. T-tube choleangiography is an examination that would be done at what point in a patient's treatment?

A. Upon admission
B. During gall bladder surgery
C. Following gall bladder surgery
D. During a gall bladder biopsy

C

1293. What is the name of the flexure that lies between the transverse colon and the descending colon?

A. Ileocecal
B. Right colic (hepatic)
C. Left colic (splenic)
D. Sigmoid

C

1294. Which of the following organs secretes insulin?

A. Pancreas
B. Adrenal
C. Duodenum
D. Ileum

A

1295. Which of the following vessels transports blood from the abdomen back to the heart?

A. Superior vena cava
B. Inferior vena cava
C. Superior mesenteric vein
D. Inferior mesenteric vein

B

1296. What percent of the population would be considered as having a sthenic body habitus?

A. 15%
B. 25%
C. 50%
D. 75%

C

1297. Which of the following structures is most distal?

A. Stomach
B. Duodenum
C. Jejunum
D. Ileum

D

1298. In this radiograph, barium was placed in the colon via which of the following routes?

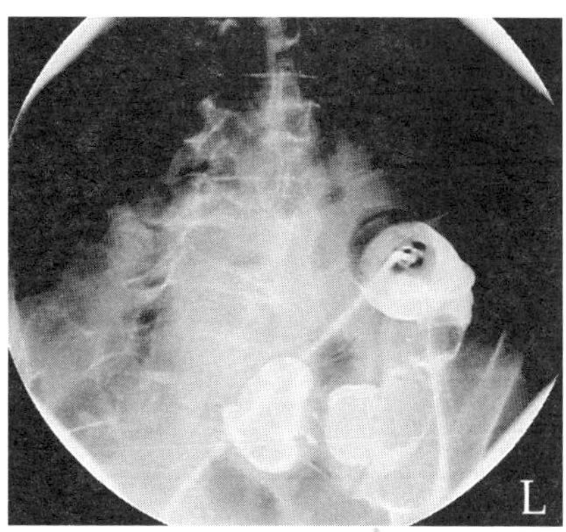

A. Rectum
B. Appendix
C. Colostomy
D. Ileum

C

1299. What is the name of the mucosal folds that are visible when the stomach is empty?

A. Haustra
B. Gastric folds
C. Omentum
D. Villi

B

1300. Which of the following radiographic procedures would routinely take the longest time to complete?

A. Colon
B. Upper GI
C. Small bowel
D. Intravenous urography

C

1301. Which of the following arteries is NOT a branch of the celiac trunk?

A. Splenic artery
B. Hepatic artery
C. Mesenteric artery
D. Left gastric artery

C

1302. What is the name of the movement that directs food down the gastrointestinal tract?

A. Peristalsis
B. Digestion
C. Deglutition
D. Mastication

A

1303. What is the membranous lining of the abdominopelvic cavity called?

A. Periosteum
B. Pleura
C. Peristalsis
D. Peritoneum

D

1304. What is the most proximal portion of the small intestine called?

A. Duodenum
B. Jejunum
C. Ileum
D. Sigmoid

A

1305. What is the name of the junction between the small intestine and the large intestine?

A. Coliointestinal junction
B. Ileocecal valve
C. Hepatocecal valve
D. Bowel articulation

B

1306. Which of the following ducts results from the union of the cystic and common hepatic ducts?

A. Gall bladder duct
B. Pancreatic duct
C. Common bile duct
D. Thoracic duct

C

1307. Which of the following are well visualized by a double-contrast barium enema?

A. Peptic ulcers
B. Colon polyps
C. G.I. bleeders
D. Hemorrhoids

B

1308. What is the outer portion of the kidney called?

A. Cortex
B. Pyramid
C. Pelvis
D. Calyx

A

1309. This double-contrast barium enema radiograph was taken with the patient in what position?

A. AP
B. RPO
C. Left lateral decubitus
D. Right lateral decubitus

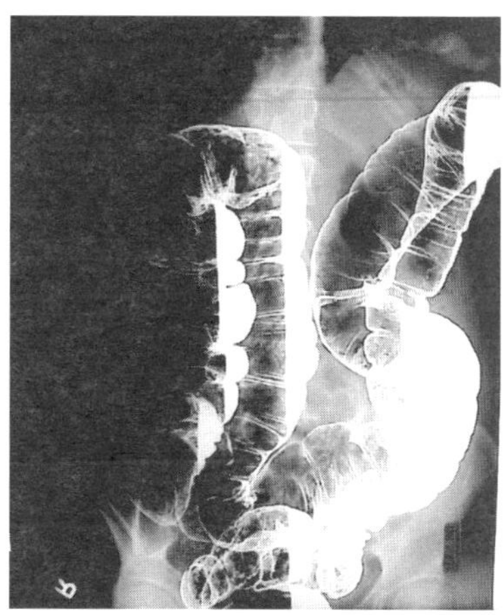

C

SKULL AND FACIAL BONES

1310. Which of the following is the part of the skull that surrounds and protects the brain?

A. Facial bones
B. Cranium
C. Foramen magnum
D. Cerebrum

B

1311. Where is the exact location of the optic foramen?

A. Base of the skull
B. Base of the orbit
C. Apex of the orbit
D. Posterior to the sella turcica

C

1312. What is the area between the eyebrows and above the bridge of the nose called?

A. Supraorbital groove
B. Nasal septum
C. Glabella
D. Calvarium

C

1313. Which of the following anatomical structures would NOT be found in the petrous portion of the temporal bone?

A. Ossicles
B. Auricle
C. Cochlea
D. Tympanic cavity

B

1314. The point where the nose and the upper lip join together is called what?

A. Acanthion
B. Nasal septum
C. Mental point
D. Alveolar process

A

1315. What is the name of the point where the two parietals articulate with the occipital bone?

A. Bregma
B. Acanthion
C. Canthus
D. Lambda

D

1316. The point where the two nasal bones and the frontal bone join together is called what?

A. Nasal septum
B. Inferior nasal conchae
C. Supraorbital groove
D. Nasion

D

1317. What is the name of the membrane that separates the external auditory meatus from the middle ear?

A. Tympanic antrum
B. Tympanic cavity
C. Tympanic membrane
D. Epitympanic recess

C

1318. What is the posterior portion of the sella turcica called?

A. Sphenoid strut
B. Dorsum sellae
C. Pituitary fossa
D. Posterior clinoid

B

1319. Which of the following facial bones are paired?

1. Vomer
2. Maxilla
3. Zygoma

A. 1 only
B. 2 only
C. 2 & 3 only
D. 1, 2 & 3

C

1320. What is the opening of the external ear canal called?

A. Auricle
B. Temporal opening
C. External auditory meatus
D. Sella turcica

C

1321. Which of the following terms describes the horizontal portion of the mandible?

A. Body
B. Ramus
C. Alveolar process
D. Condyloid process

A

1322. A line drawn between the two pupils of the eyes defines which of the positioning lines?

A. Interpupillary line
B. Intercanthus line
C. Biorbital line
D. Base line

A

1323. What is the name of the canal that connects the nasopharynx with the middle ear?

A. Auditory canal
B. Internal auditory canal
C. Nasal cavity
D. Eustachian tube

D

1324. If the orbitomeatal line was perpendicular to the image receptor for the PA (Caldwell) projection to the right, how was the CR angled?

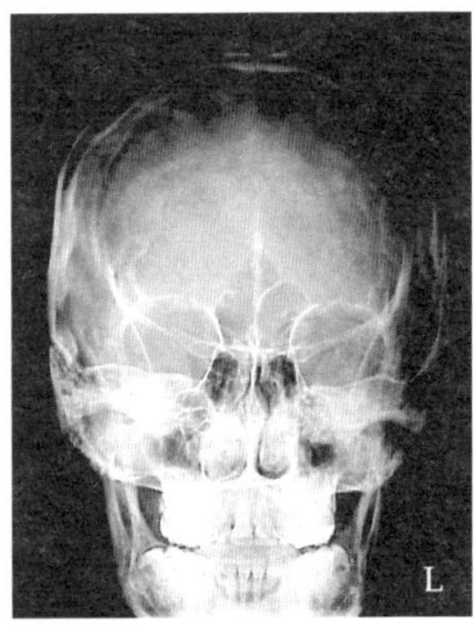

A. 15^0 caudad
B. 15^0 cephalad
C. 30^0 caudad
D. 30^0 cephalad

A

1325. A line drawn between the lateral margin of the orbit and the E.A.M. is called what?

A. Glabellomeatal line
B. Orbitomeatal line
C. Outer orbital line
D. External meatal line

B

1326. Which of the following projections are taken to demonstrate the temporomandibular joints?

A. PA and parietoacanthial (Waters) projection
B. Open and closed mouth lateral (Law) projection
C. PA (Caldwell) projection and parietoacanthial (Waters) projection
D. Axiolateral (Mayers) projection and posterior profile (Stenvers) projection

B

1327. Which of the following is considered the master gland of the endocrine system?

A. Pineal
B. Pituitary
C. Pancreas
D. Parotid

B

1328. What is the line called between the infraorbital margin and the E.A.M. called?

A. Infraorbitomeatal line
B. Canthomeatal line
C. Infraorbital line
D. Glabellomeatal line

A

1329. Which of the following would be an alternate projection for a patient who cannot flex his/her neck sufficiently for an AP axial (Towne) projection?

A. AP (Caldwell) projection
B. AP (Fuchs) projection
C. Axiolateral (Schuller) projection
D. PA axial (Haas) projection

D

1330. A line between the acanthion and the external auditory meatus is known as what?

A. Glabellomeatal line
B. Mentomeatal line
C. Alveolar line
D. Acanthiomeatal line

D

1331. For a parietoacanthial (Waters) projection, the patient is instructed to rest his/her head on which of the following?

A. Nose
B. Cheek
C. Chin
D. Forehead

C

1332. What is the superior most aspect of the skull called?

A. Floor
B. Calvarium
C. Vertex
D. Cranium

C

1333. Which of the following projections will demonstrate both zygomatic arches?

A. Submentovertical (full basal) projection
B. Axiolateral
C. Biparietal
D. Axial oblique

A

1334. Which of the following topographical landmarks corresponds to the floor of the cranium?

A. Supraorbital groove
B. Interpupillary line
C. Mental point
D. E.A.M.

A

1335. For a true lateral position of the skull, the midsagittal plane must be in which of these positions?

A. Perpendicular to the image receptor
B. Parallel to the image receptor
C. At a right angle to the image receptor
D. Parallel to the central ray

B

1336. What is another name for the posterior angle of the mandible?

A. Inion
B. Gonion
C. Pinna
D. Mental point

B

1337. Which of the following glands will be demonstrated if contrast media is injected into Stensen's duct?

A. Submandibular
B. Sublingual
C. Pineal
D. Parotid

D

1338. What is the correct anatomical term describing the skull cap?

A. Calvarium
B. Cranium
C. Vertex
D. Parietals

A

1339. The perpendicular plate of the ethmoid bone articulates with which of the following facial bones?

A. Maxilla
B. Zygoma
C. Vomer
D. Palatine

C

1340. Which of the following is NOT one of the bones that composes the calvarium?

A. Frontal
B. Temporal
C. Occipital
D. Parietal

B

1341. How many salivary glands are there?

A. 2
B. 4
C. 6
D. 8

C

1342. What suture separates the two parietal bones?

A. Coronal
B. Lambdoidal
C. Sagittal
D. Squamosal

C

1343. What is the flat, major part of the parietal bone called?

A. Petrous portion
B. Squamous portion
C. Sagittal portion
D. Temporal portion

B

1344. Which line should be perpendicular to the plane of the image receptor for a true lateral skull position?

A Infraorbitomeatal line
B. Orbitomeatal line
C. Acanthiomeatal line
D. Interpupillary line

D

1345. Which of the following will best be demonstrated with a submentovertical (full basal) projection of the skull?

A. Orbits
B. Mandible
C. Base of cranium
D. Frontal sinuses

C

1346. Which of the following is a reliable way to check for rotation on a lateral skull radiograph?

A. Mandibular rami superimposed
B. Sella turcica visualized
C. Cranial floor superimposed
D. E.A.M. superimposed on mastoid tip

A

1347. The cribriform plate is a part of which of these bones?

A. Frontal
B. Sphenoid
C. Ethmoid
D. Vomer

C

1348. If the orbitomeatal line is perpendicular to the image receptor for an AP axial (Towne) projection, how much caudal angle is required?

A. 25^0
B. 30^0
C. 37^0
D. 40^0

B

1349. The orbitomeatal line is perpendicular to the image receptor and the CR is angled 15^0 cephalic. What projection is this?

A. PA (Caldwell) projection
B. AP (Caldwell) projection
C. AP axial (Towne) projection
D. Submentovertical (full basal) projection

B

1350. Which of the following is NOT one of the auditory ossicles?

A. Incus
B. Stapes
C. Malleus
D. Meatus

D

1351. Why is the radiograph to the right NOT an acceptable parietoacanthial (Waters) projection?

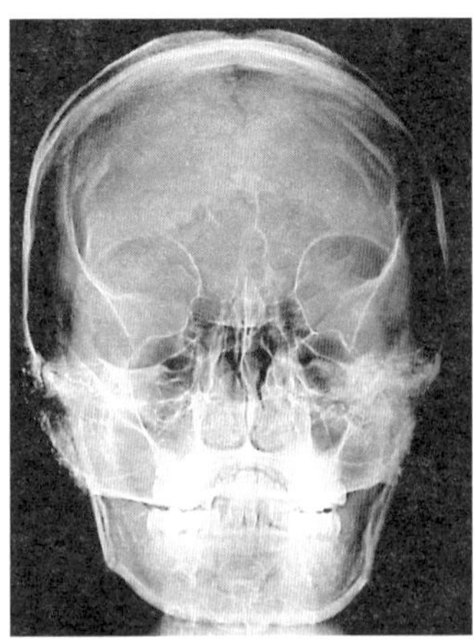

A. The skull is rotated
B. The orbits are magnified
C. The frontal sinuses are not visualized
D. The petrous ridges are not projected directly below the maxillary sinuses

D

1352. For a submentovertical (full basal) projection, what line is parallel to the plane of the image receptor?

A. Glabellomeatal line
B. Orbitomeatal line
C. Infraorbitomeatal line
D. Acanthiomeatal line

C

1353. For the lateral (Law) projection of the TMJ's, how much is the central ray angled and in which direction?

A. 15^0 cephalad
B. 15^0 caudad
C. 30^0 cephalad
D. 30^0 caudad

B

1354. What two parts of the patient's anatomy will be touching the table during a PA (Caldwell) projection?

A. Nose and chin
B. Nose and forehead
C. Upper and lower lips
D. Cheek and chin

B

1355. Which of the following projections would demonstrate the facial bones and the zygomatic arches?

A. Parietoacanthial (Waters) projection
B. PA (Caldwell) projection
C. AP axial (Towne) projection
D. Submentovertical (full basal) projection

A

1356. What structure should be projected within the shadow of the foramen magnum on a well positioned AP axial (Towne) projection of the skull?

A. Petrous pyramids
B. Inion
C. Dorsum sellae
D. Posterior cervical arch

C

1357. For an axiolateral oblique projection of the mandible, if the patient is lateral, how much is the tube angled?

A. 15^0 cephalad
B. 25^0 cephalad
C. 35^0 cephalad
D. 45^0 cephalad

B

1358. If the foramen magnum is NOT well visualized on an AP axial (Towne) projection radiograph of the skull, what must be done to correct it?

A. Increase CR angle caudally
B. Decrease CR angle caudally
C. Eliminate CR angle
D. Orbitomeatal line is parallel

A

1359. What is the name of the bony plate that divides the nasal cavity?

A. Nasal ridge
B. Nasal septum
C. Nasal spine
D. Nasal bone

B

1360. Where will the petrous pyramids be projected in a properly positioned PA (Caldwell) projection radiograph?

A. In the center of the orbits
B. In the upper 1/3 of the orbits
C. In the lower 1/3 of the orbits
D. In the lower 1/8 of the orbits

C

1361. What is the name of the structure that houses the pituitary gland?

A. Sella turcica
B. Sphenoid strut
C. Sphenoid fossa
D. Turk's fossa

A

1362. What structure must be entirely in front of (anterior to) both petrous pyramids on a submentovertical (full basal) radiograph of the skull?

A. Mandible
B. Floor of the cranium
C. Foramen magnum
D. Sella turcica

A

1363. Which of the following is NOT a facial bone?

A. Maxilla
B. Mandible
C. Lacrimal
D. Ethmoid

D

1364. Which position/projection would be used to best demonstrate the frontal bone?

A. PA (Caldwell) projection
B. AP axial (Towne) projection
C. Submentovertical (full basal) projection
D. Lateral

A

1365. Which of the following positions/projections will best demonstrate a "blow-out" fracture of the orbit?

A. Lateral
B. Parietoacanthial (Waters) projection
C. PA (modified Waters) projection
D. PA (Caldwell) projection

C

1366. Which position/projection would be used to best demonstrate the occipital bone?

A. PA (Caldwell) projection
B. AP axial (Towne) projection
C. Submentovertical (full basal) projection
D. Lateral

B

1367. Which of the following bones helps form the base of the cranium?

A. Sphenoid
B. Parietal
C. Occipital
D. Frontal

A

1368. To best demonstrate the floor of the cranium, which position/projection would be used?

A. Lateral
B. AP axial (Towne) projection
C. Submentovertical (full basal) projection
D. PA (Caldwell) projection

C

1369. The tear ducts are associated with which of the following bones?

A. Nasal
B. Ethmoid
C. Lacrimal
D. Maxilla

C

1370. If the CR enters at a point 3/4" anterior and 3/4" superior to the E.A.M., what structure would be visualized?

A. Petrous pyramid
B. Foramen magnum
C. Floor of the cranium
D. Sella turcica

D

1371. What are the names of the "L" shaped bones that are located posterior to the nasal cavity?

A. Nasal conchae
B. Palatine
C. Maxilla
D. Zygomatic

B

1372. The bregma in an adult would be referred to as what in an infant?

A. Anterior fontanel
B. Posterior fontanel
C. Anterior fissure
D. Posterior sulcus

A

1373. Where should the central ray enter for a cross table lateral, trauma skull projection?

A. Perpendicular to the EAM
B. 3/4" anterior and 3/4" superior to the EAM
C. 2" superior to the EAM
D. The lateral margin of the orbit

C

1374. Which of the following articulates with the zygomatic bones?

A. Nasal
B. Lacrimal
C. Temporal
D. Mandible

C

1375. Which of the following areas would have to be radiographed in order to demonstrate the sphenoid strut?

A. Base of the cranium
B. Sella turcica
C. Middle ear
D. Orbit

D

1376. What is the name of the part of the temporal bone that houses the organs of hearing and equilibrium?

A. Petrous
B. Squamous
C. Mastoid
D. Alveolar

A

1377. For an AP 0 degree (Caldwell) projection of a trauma skull, where will the central ray enter?

A. Acanthion
B. Glabella
C. Nasion
D. Forehead

B

1378. Which of the following bones does NOT help form the base of the orbit?

A. Frontal
B. Maxilla
C. Zygoma
D. Nasal

D

1379. Which of the following is NOT one of the sutures of the cranium?

A. Coronal
B. Squamosal
C. Lambdoidal
D. Occipital

D

1380. Of the following radiographic projections, which one will show all of the paranasal sinuses?

A. PA
B. Parietoacanthial (Waters) projection
C. Lateral
D. Submentovertical (full basal) projection

C

1381. Where does the central ray exit for a parietoacanthial (Waters) projection of the facial bones?

A. Acanthion
B. Nasion
C. Glabella
D. Inner canthus

A

1382. For a posterior profile (Stenvers) projection of the temporal bone, how does the head rest on the radiographic table?

A. Forehead, cheek and chin
B. Forehead, cheek and nose
C. Forehead, nose and chin
D. Nose, cheek and chin

B

1383. For a lateral (Schuller) projection of the TMJ's, how is the central ray angled?

A. 12^0 cephalad
B. 12^0 caudad
C. 25^0 cephalad
D. 25^0 caudad

D

1384. In order to demonstrate fluid in the sinuses, the patient must be radiographed in which position?

A. Supine
B. Prone
C. Erect
D. Trendelenburg

C

1385. What position is obtained if the head is in a lateral position and the central ray enters the zygoma?

A. Lateral facial bones
B. Lateral paranasal sinuses
C. Lateral skull
D. Lateral mandible

A

1386. How is the tube angled for a posterior profile (Stenvers) projection of the temporal bone?

A. 12^0 cephalad
B. 12^0 caudad
C. 20^0 cephalad
D. 20^0 caudad

A

1387. A radiographic examination of the nasal bones would consist of which of the following positions/projections?

A. Parietoacanthial (Waters) projection and lateral
B. Parietoacanthial (Waters) projection and PA (Caldwell) projection
C. Parietoacanthial (Waters) projection and both laterals
D. Parietoacanthial (Waters) projection, AP axial (Towne) projection and lateral

C

1388. What is the name of the bony ridge that lies beneath the eyebrows?

A. Glabella
B. Supercilliary ridge
C. Supraorbital groove
D. Anterior orbital protuberance

B

1389. What is the name of the small gland that lies in the midline of the brain and is often calcified in the adult?

A. Pineal
B. Pituitary
C. Thyroid
D. Parathyroid

A

1390. Which of the following bones forms the major part of the hard palate?

A. Palatines
B. Maxillae
C. Zygomatics
D. Mandible

B

1391. What is the name of the large opening in the base of the cranium through which the spinal cord passes?

A. Optic foramen
B. Foramen ovale
C. Foramen lacerum
D. Foramen magnum

D

CHAPTER FIVE

PATIENT CARE

- General Patient Care (64 questions)
- Aseptic and Isolation Techniques (38 questions)
- Vital Signs and Drugs (30 questions)
- Basic Medical Terminology (36 questions)
- Circulatory and Skeletal Diseases (54 questions)
- Digestive and Urinary Diseases (34 questions)
- Respiratory and Other Diseases (54 questions)
- Venipuncture (25 questions)

1392. Which of the following would describe an ambulatory patient?

A. One that is bedridden
B. One that cannot speak
C. One that is able to walk
D. One that arrived by ambulance

C

1393. Which of the following conditions would be considered "hard to penetrate"?

A. Emphysema
B. Osteoporosis
C. Osteosclerosis
D. Pneumothorax

C

1394. Which of the following may cause a patient to faint?

1. Hunger
2. Emotional stress
3. Lack of sleep

A. 1 only
B. 1 & 2 only
C. 1 & 3 only
D. 1, 2 & 3

D

1395. Which of the following should be done when moving a patient with a broken arm?

A. Support only the elbow
B. Support only the wrist
C. Support the entire arm
D. Support only the forearm

C

1396. A radiographer's primary responsibility is to which of the following?

A. The radiologist
B. The patient's needs
C. The hospital
D. The radiology department

B

1397. Which of the following describes a paraplegic?

A. Paralyzed from the waist up
B. Paralyzed from the waist down
C. Paralyzed on one side
D. Paralyzed in all four extremities

B

1398. If someone needs to hold a patient during a radiographic procedure, who should be asked?

A. A student
B. A nurse's aide
C. Another technologist
D. The patient's family member

D

1399. The patient in insulin shock who is still conscious requires which of the following?

A. Something with sugar
B. Something salty
C. More insulin
D. An immediate transfusion

A

1400. What is the proper procedure for turning a disabled patient on an x-ray table?

A. Turn the patient away from you
B. Turn the patient's legs first
C. Turn the patient toward you
D. Turn the patient whichever way is easier

C

1401. Which of the following would be considered an unethical practice for a radiographer?

A. Repeating a radiograph
B. Watching an interesting case
C. Criticizing a doctor or team member
D. Reporting unethical practices

C

1402. During a myelogram, what position is the patient in when his head is put lower than his feet?

A. Fowler
B. Prone
C. Trendelenburg
D. Sim's

C

1403. Which of the following is the rule for pediatric patients undergoing a radiographic exam?

A. Always restrain children
B. Never restrain children
C. Restrain children under 2 years old
D. Restrain children when necessary

D

1404. A professional assessment of a patient's health will require which of the following?

1. Observe his physical condition
2. Note his mental state
3. Be aware of his cultural background

A. 1 only
B. 1 & 2 only
C. 2 & 3 only
D. 1, 2 & 3

D

1405. Which of the following cannot be done when in the same room with a patient receiving oxygen?

A. Smoke
B. Talk
C. Bring in plants
D. Bring in portable x-ray equipment

A

1406. What is the correct order for administering basic life support?

A. Circulation, breathing, airway
B. Airway, circulation, breathing
C. Breathing, circulation, airway
D. Airway, breathing, circulation

D

1407. When the body is invaded by pathogens, what is the response in the bloodstream?

A Red blood cells increase
B. White blood cells increase
C. DNA increases
D. Serum increases

B

1408. Which of the following elements are currently found in all intravenous solutions of contrast media?

A. Iodine
B. Nitrogen
C. Sulfur
D. Barium

A

1409. If you determine that a patient is in need of CPR, what should be your first response?

A. Begin cardiac compressions
B. Run for help
C. Begin mouth to mouth
D. Call for help

D

1410. If a patient has an allergic reaction to the contrast media during an IVU, which should be done first?

A. Apply cold compresses
B. Inject 5 cc's of Benadryl
C. Inject 5 ml's of adrenalin
D. Call for a doctor

D

1411. What is the most severe form of convulsive seizures?

A. Petit mal
B. Grand mal
C. Partial
D. Epileptic

B

1412. When lifting a patient, what must you remember?

1. Keep your back straight
2. Keep your arms straight
3. Keep your legs straight

A. 1 only
B. 2 only
C. 1 & 3 only
D. 1, 2 & 3

A

1413. If CPR is NOT started within _____ of cardiac arrest, there will be brain damage due to lack of oxygen.

A. 1-3 minutes
B. 4-6 minutes
C. 7-10 minutes
D. 15 minutes

A

1414. Which of the following diseases is NOT considered communicable?

A. Pneumonia
B. Tuberculosis
C. Gastritis
D. Hepatitis

C

1415. While in an operating room, what precautions can be taken to minimize the explosive hazard?

1. Clean the x-ray equipment
2. Wear covers over shoes
3. Wear caps over head

A. 1 & 2 only
B. 1 & 3 only
C. 2 & 3 only
D. 1, 2 & 3

D

1416. What is the type of shock that is caused by a failure of the heart to pump enough blood to the vital organs?

A. Cardiogenic shock
B. Septic shock
C. Anaphylactic shock
D. Hypovolemic shock

A

1417. What should be your first action if a patient is bleeding profusely from an open leg wound?

A. Go for a nurse
B. Apply direct pressure to the wound
C. Go for a doctor
D. Finish the radiographs quickly

B

1418. If a patient convulses in the x-ray department, the radiographer should do which of the following?

A. Insert a padded tongue blade
B. Restrain the patient
C. Prevent injury to the patient
D. Put the patient on the floor

C

1419. Which of the following needles has the smallest lumen?

A. 15 gauge
B. 19 gauge
C. 21 gauge
D. 25 gauge

D

1420. If a patient's I.V. site becomes puffy and swollen, what should the radiographer do?

A. Pull the needle out and restart the I.V.
B. Check with the head nurse
C. Clamp off the I.V.
D. Do nothing

C

1421. A written page or spoken word are examples of which of the following components of communication?

A. Message
B. Channel
C. Source
D. Feedback

B

1422. While in the operating room, which of the following is NOT considered a sterile area?

A. The patient
B. An instrument table
C. The anesthetist
D. A scrub nurse

C

1423. An unconscious patient whose skin is dry and has a fruity odor on his/her breath is a classic example of what?

A. Drunkenness
B. Insulin shock
C. Diabetes
D. Diabetic coma

D

1424. What does it mean to administer drugs parenterally?

1. I.V. or by injection
2. Orally
3. Rectally

A. 1 only
B. 2 only
C. 2 & 3 only
D. 1, 2 & 3

A

1425. For a patient with I.V. therapy, how high above the vein should the container of solution be kept?

A. As high as possible
B. 10-12"
C. 18-20"
D. 28-30"

C

1426. Which of the following would NOT be used in restraining a child?

A. A sheet
B. A leather belt
C. A pillow case
D. Sandbags

B

1427. The "threat of touching a person in a harmful manner" is the legal definition of what?

A. Assault
B. Battery
C. Injury
D. Negligence

A

1428. Which of the following conditions would be considered "easy to penetrate"?

A. Edema
B. Degenerative arthritis
C. Paget's disease
D. Pneumonia

B

1429. Which of the following is an example of good body mechanics?

A. Bend from the knees
B. Keep feet close together
C. Bend from the waist
D. Carry objects at arms length

A

1430. What type of shock is caused by loss of blood due to a knife or gunshot wound?

A. Cardiogenic shock
B. Septic shock
C. Anaphylactic shock
D. Hypovolemic shock

D

1431. Which of the following best describes the Fowler position?

A. Head lower than feet
B. Feet lower than head
C. Prone
D. Lateral recumbent

B

1432. According to Maslow's hierarchy, which of the following is a person's most basic need?

A. Safety and security
B. Self-esteem
C. Physiological needs
D. Self-actualization

C

1433. What stage of grieving is the terminally ill patient in when he/she begins to deal with his/her pain and illness?

A. Depression stage
B. Acceptance stage
C. Anger stage
D. Bargaining stage

B

1434. Which of the following would be considered an example of negative non-verbal communication?

A. A smile
B. Eye contact
C. Leaning toward patient when talking
D. Standing with your arms crossed

D

1435. Which of the following procedures would require an informed consent form to be completed?

A. Upper G.I. series
B. Cerebral angiogram
C. T-tube choleangiogram
D. Barium enema

B

1436. While radiographing a patient with chest tube drainage, which of the following actions must be taken?

A. Clamp drainage tube
B. Keep drainage tube below chest
C. Raise drainage system above chest
D. Turn pump off during the exam

B

1437. What can happen if a diabetic patient has taken his/her normal dose of insulin but has been NPO since midnight?

A. Go into diabetic coma
B. Go into insulin shock
C. Develop difficulty breathing
D. Dehydrate

B

1438. A patient in a diabetic coma needs which of the following?

A. Something with sugar
B. Something salty
C. More insulin
D. An immediate transfusion

C

1439. What is the best way to move a heavy object, such as a case of x-ray film?

A. Hold it away from your body
B. Push it
C. Drag it
D. Lift it up

B

1440. How should you have an ambulatory patient get off the radiographic table?

A. Use a footstool
B. Jump to the floor
C. Get on a stretcher
D. Get in a wheelchair

A

1441. What is the best way to make sure that you have the correct patient for a radiographic examination?

A. Call the patient's name
B. Take the next patient in line
C. Check the patient's armband
D. Ask the receptionist who is next

C

1442. Which of the following sites would be best for I.V. therapy?

A. The leg
B. The arm
C. The neck
D. The foot

B

1443. What is the usual rate of flow for an adult with an I.V. in use?

A. 2 drops per minute
B. 20 drops per minute
C. 60 drops per minute
D. 99 drops per minute

D

1444. "Touching a patient without permission" is the legal definition of what?

A. Assault
B. Malpractice
C. Battery
D. Perjury

C

1445. When transferring a patient from a wheelchair to the x-ray table which action would you do first?

A. Lock the wheelchair brakes
B. Raise footrests out of the way
C. Put wheelchair parallel to the table
D. Help patient to stand

C

1446. When inserting an enema tip, what position is the patient in?

A. Fowler
B. Prone
C. Trendelenburg
D. Sim's

D

1447. Where should a patient's urinary bag be kept while transferring him/her from the stretcher to the x-ray table?

A. Resting on the patient's legs
B. Below bladder level
C. At bladder level
D. Between the stretcher and table

B

1448. According to Elizabeth Kubler Ross, what is the first stage of the grieving process?

A. Bargaining
B. Acceptance
C. Denial
D. Anger

C

1449. Which of the following is NOT a legal right of a patient in the radiology department?

A. To know the technologist's name
B. To refuse the radiographic exam
C. To be informed of the possible risks
D. To ask for and receive extra studies

D

1450. What is the most common work-related problem among health care workers?

A. Infection due to patient contact
B. Excessive radiation exposure
C. Diseases from dirty needles
D. Back problems from improper lifting

D

1451. When radiographing a number of patients in a row, you should do which of the following?

A. Avoid using a pillow
B. Change the pillowcase after each use
C. Change the linen twice a day
D. Do not worry about changing linen

B

1452. What is the first thing you should do if a patient who is standing turns pale and says he feels dizzy?

A. Quickly make the exposure
B. Have the patient inhale ammonia
C. Take the patient's blood pressure
D. Have the patient lie down

D

1453. What type of shock can result from a severe reaction to the contrast media used in radiographic exams?

A. Hypovolemic shock
B. Septic shock
C. Anaphylactic shock
D. Cardiogenic shock

C

1454. A patient with a head injury should be kept in which of the following positions?

A. Erect
B. Semi-erect
C. Supine
D. Trendelenburg

B

1455. When is an I.V. considered to be infiltrated?

A. When blood is seen in I.V. tubing
B. When the needle is accidently pulled out
C. When solution is leaking into tissue
D. When the I.V. is injected into

C

ASEPTIC AND ISOLATION TECHNIQUES

1456. What is the definition of a fomite?

A. An insect
B. A method of sterilization
C. A small animal
D. An item to which microorganisms cling

D

1457. Which of the following is NOT a method of sterilization?

A. Chemicals
B. Dry heat
C. Steam under pressure
D. Handwashing

D

1458. By what method are pathogens spread when a person coughs or sneezes?

A. Vector
B. Vehicle
C. Direct contact
D. Droplet

D

1459. What should be done with a plastic cassette cover after it is used to cover a cassette during an isolation patient's exam?

A. Take it with you
B. Leave it on the floor in the isolation room
C. Discard it in a red, infectious waste, plastic bag
D. Use it for the next isolation patient

C

1460. The establishment and growth of microorganisms on or in a host defines which of the following?

A. Pathogen
B. Infection
C. Disease
D. Bacteria

B

1461. Which of the following is an example of a fomite?

A. An insect
B. A method of sterilization
C. A small animal
D. A radiographic cassette

D

1462. The complete removal of all microorganisms from an object is called what?

A. Antiseptic
B. Medical asepsis
C. Sterile technique
D. Sterilization

D

1463. When a disease is spread by an insect depositing the pathogens on or in a human, it is transmitted by what method?

A. Vector
B. Vehicle
C. Direct contact
D. Droplet

A

1464. Sterilization in an autoclave involves which of the following?

A. Chemicals
B. Steam under pressure
C. Dry heat
D. Ionizing radiation

B

1465. If you come across a sterile tray that has no expiration date on it, what should you do?

A. Use it immediately
B. Use it within a week
C. Consider it unsterile
D. Consider it sterile

C

1466. The Centers of Disease Control (CDC) recommends that all health care providers:

1. wear gloves when touching blood, body fluids or broken skin of all patients.
2. wash hands immediately if they become contaminated with blood or other body fluids.
3. place syringes, needles, and sharp items in puncture-resistant containers for disposal.

A. 1 & 2 only
B. 1 & 3 only
C. 2 & 3 only
D. 1, 2 & 3

D

1467. A disease spread by kissing is being transmitted by which of the following methods?

A. Direct contact
B. Vector
C. Droplet
D. Vehicle

A

1468. Which of the following is necessary when doing a portable chest radiograph on a patient on droplet precautions?

A. Wearing a mask
B. Wearing a gown
C. Wearing gloves
D. A ventilated room

A

1469. The CDC has revised the isolation precautions to clarify confusing terms such as universal precautions and body substance isolation. What is the new terminology?

A. Personnel precautions
B. Protective isolation
C. Standard precautions
D. Isolation techniques

C

1470. While in a sterile gown, the sterile field is considered to end where?

A. At the level of your shoulders
B. At the hem of the gown
C. At the level of your hands
D. At the waist of the gown

D

1471. How should two people in sterile gowns pass each other?

A. Front to front
B. Back to back
C. Right side to right side
D. Right side to left side

B

1472. In opening a cloth-wrapped sterile pack, how should the first outer corner be opened?

A. With sterile gloves
B. Towards you
C. Away from you
D. To the side

C

1473. Which of the following would be appropriate when a sterile gown must be worn during fluoroscopy?

A. Lead apron worn backward
B. Lead apron cannot be worn
C. Lead apron worn under the gown
D. Lead apron worn over the gown

C

1474. Which of the following parts of a sterile gown are considered sterile?

A. Below the waist in front
B. The sleeves
C. Below the waist in back
D. The back

B

1475. If a patient is known to be infected with a pathogenic organism or communicable disease which of the following is applied?

A. Isolation precautions
B. Reverse isolation
C. Personal precautions
D. Transmission-based precautions

D

1476. A disease spread through contaminated water or food is being transmitted by which of the following methods?

A. Vector
B. Vehicle
C. Direct contact
D. Droplet

B

1477. How should the scrub be performed when preparing a patient's skin for a special procedure?

A. From the center out
B. From the outside in
C. Right to left
D. Top to bottom

A

1478. When painting a patient's skin for a special procedure, how many passes should be made with the same sponge?

A. One
B. Two
C. Three
D. Four

A

1479. Which of the following organs is sterile?

A. Stomach
B. Urinary bladder
C. Large intestine
D. Pharynx

B

1480. Which of the following terms is best defined as any disease producing microorganism?

A. Pathogen
B. Fungus
C. Bacterium
D. Asepsis

A

1481. An infection that the patient acquires while in the hospital is known as what?

A. Viral infection
B. Gangrenous infection
C. Nosocomial infection
D. Hospitality infection

C

1482. Which of the following classifications do yeasts and molds fit into?

A. Viruses
B. Fungi
C. Bacteria
D. Pathologies

B

1483. Which of the following is the most effective method for achieving medical asepsis?

A. Frequent handwashing
B. Having employees in perfect health
C. Changing linen after every patient
D. Cleaning the x-ray table often

A

1484. The common cold is an example of a disease process caused by which of the following?

1. Virus
2. Bacterium
3. Fungus

A. 1 only
B. 2 only
C. 1 & 3 only
D. 1, 2 & 3

A

1485. Staphylococci and bacilli are classified as what type of microorganisms?

A. Viruses
B. Bacteria
C. Fungi
D. Molds

B

1486. Medical asepsis is the _______ of microorganisms in the immediate environment.

A. Complete destruction and removal
B. Method of encouraging growth
C. Method of creating new types
D. Reduction without sterilization

D

1487. What should be done with the portable unit after doing an isolation patient with a respiratory disease?

A. It must be sterilized
B. It must be wiped with a disinfectant
C. It cannot be used for 24 hours
D. Nothing needs to be done

B

1488. Which of the following is necessary before entering the operating room with a portable radiographic unit?

1. The portable unit must be wiped with a disinfectant
2. The technologist must be masked, gowned and gloved
3. The portable unit must be wiped free of dust

A. 1 only
B. 2 only
C. 3 only
D. 2 & 3 only

A

1489. Which of the following diseases is NOT considered communicable?

A. Hepatitis
B. Mononucleosis
C. Pneumonia
D. Gastritis

D

1490. How should used needles be disposed of?

A. Placed, uncapped, in a red sharps container
B. Placed, recapped, in a red sharps container
C. Placed, recapped, in a red trash bag
D. Placed, uncapped, in a red trash bag

A

1491. Which of the following must be followed when pouring solutions into a container on a sterile tray?

1. Hold the solution well above the tray
2. Prevent the solution from splashing
3. Prevent drips from landing on the tray

A. 1 & 2 only
B. 1 & 3 only
C. 2 & 3 only
D. 1, 2 & 3

D

1492. What is the greatest hazard in the operating room?

A. Explosion
B. Contamination
C. Electrical shock
D. Cardiogenic shock

B

1493. Which of the following must be done with the cassettes after they are used for an isolation patient?

A. Destroyed
B. Set aside for 24 hours
C. Disinfected before put in the darkroom
D. Left in the pillowcase

C

1494. Which of the following is NOT a reliable method for taking a person's temperature?

A. Orally
B. Rectally
C. On the forehead
D. In the axilla

C

1495. Nitroglycerin is used medically as which of the following?

A. A vasoconstrictor
B. An anesthetic
C. An analgesic
D. A vasodilator

D

1496. What is the name of a vein in the antecubital space that is often used as an injection site for an IVU?

A. Ulnar vein
B. Humeral vein
C. Radial vein
D. Basilic vein

D

1497. What is the normal range of diastolic pressure for adults?

A. 40-80 mm Hg
B. 60-90 mm Hg
C. 80-120 mm Hg
D. 110-140 mm Hg

B

1498. What is a normal respiratory rate for an adult?

A. 8-12 respirations per minute
B. 12-16 respirations per minute
C. 16-20 respirations per minute
D. 25-30 respirations per minute

B

1499. In most cases, if the patient's blood pressure is high, then their pulse rate will be what?

A. Rapid
B. Slow
C. Normal
D. Zero

B

1500. What type of drug is penicillin?

A. Antihistamine
B. Anticoagulant
C. Antibiotic
D. Vasoconstrictor

C

1501. What type of drug is Dilantin?

A. Anticoagulant
B. Antiepileptic
C. Antihistamine
D. Antiheart failure medication

B

1502. What is the most accurate method for taking a temperature?

A. The rectal method
B. The oral method
C. In the axilla
D. On the forehead

A

1503. What is the average pulse rate of an infant?

A. 30-40 beats per minute
B. 50-60 beats per minute
C. 70-80 beats per minute
D. 115-130 beats per minute

D

1504. Which of the following is the normal range for oral temperatures?

A. 97-98 degrees
B. 98-99 degrees
C. 96-100 degrees
D. 99-100 degrees

B

1505. A patient's temperature taken rectally is usually what?

A. 1 degree higher than orally
B. 1 degree lower than orally
C. 2 degrees higher than orally
D. 2 degrees lower than orally

A

1506. Epinephrine is what type of drug?

A. Antibiotic
B. Bronchodilator
C. Anesthetic
D. Antiarrhythmic

B

1507. Which of the following drugs is an anticoagulant?

A. Demerol
B. Heparin
C. Benadryl
D. Penicillin

B

1508. When a shot is given into the upper arm or buttocks, how is it being administered?

A. IM
B. IV
C. Subcutaneous
D. Intraspinal

A

1509. What is a sphygmomanometer used for?

A. Delivering oxygen
B. Administering medication
C. Restraining a patient
D. Taking blood pressure

D

1510. Demerol is what type of drug?

A. Respiratory stimulant
B. Local anesthetic
C. Analgesic
D. Antibiotic

C

1511. Benadryl is associated with the treatment of which of the following?

A. Vomiting
B. Allergies
C. Hypotension
D. Epilepsy

B

1512. Which of the following blood pressures would indicate hypertension?

1. 140/70
2. 140/90
3. 120/99

A. 1 only
B. 3 only
C. 1 & 3 only
D. 1, 2 & 3

B

1513. A patient's blood pressure is 120/78. What does the figure 120 represent?

A. Systolic pressure
B. High blood pressure
C. Diastolic pressure
D. Pressure of ventricular relaxation

A

1514. Which of the following conditions can be treated with the drug Aminophylline?

A. Heart failure
B. Epilepsy
C. Cancer
D. Asthma

D

1515. Digoxin is associated with the treatment of which of the following?

A. Cancer
B. Barbiturate poisoning
C. Heart failure
D. Asthma

C

1516. In order to see a very quick effect of a drug, how should it be administered?

A. Intramuscularly
B. Intravenously
C. Orally
D. Subcutaneously

B

1517. Your patient indicates he needs nitroglycerin for his angina. How should it be administered?

A. Rectally
B. Orally
C. Intravenously
D. Sublingually

D

1518. Which of the following methods of administering a drug would NOT be considered parenteral?

A. Oral
B. Intravenous
C. Intramuscular
D. Subcutaneous

A

1519. What type of drug is Benadryl?

A. Antihistamine
B. Vasodilator
C. Anticoagulant
D. Anesthetic

A

1520. Which of the following drugs is synonymous with Adrenaline?

A. Benadryl
B. Nitroglycerin
C. Epinephrine
D. Heparin

C

1521. When performing CPR on an adult, with another person, which of the following must be followed?

A. 2 respirations then 5 compressions
B. 5 respirations then 10 compressions
C. 2 respirations then 15 compressions
D. 5 respirations then 30 compressions

C

1522. What is the average pulse rate for an adult?

A. 30-40 beats per minute
B. 50-60 beats per minute
C. 70-80 beats per minute
D. 90-99 beats per minute

C

1523. What is the normal range for systolic pressure in an adult?

A. 40-80 mm Hg
B. 60-70 mm Hg
C. 80-120 mm Hg
D. 110-140 mm Hg

D

BASIC MEDICAL TERMINOLOGY

1524. Which of the following abbreviations means to provide medication "whenever necessary"?

A. q.h.
B. pid
C. qid
D. prn

D

1525. Which of the following refers to a test that records the brain waves?

A. EEG
B. EKG
C. ECG
D. BWG

A

1526. Which of the following may describe a patient's heart attack?

A. MI
B. HA
C. CVA
D. CPR

A

1527. "Rx" is the abbreviation for which of the following?

A. Diagnosis
B. Prescription
C. Fracture
D. Respiration

B

1528. Which of the following abbreviations means to provide medication "4 times a day"?

A. qid
B. prn
C. q4hr
D. qh

A

1529. An abbreviation meaning a "stroke" is which of the following?

A. EEG
B. CHF
C. CVA
D. SOB

C

1530. The abbreviation "BUN" stands for what?

A. Bad ureteral nick
B. Bloody urine nephron
C. Blood urea nitrogen
D. Brain underlying necrosis

C

1531. What is another term for bleeding?

A. Abrasion
B. Hemorrhage
C. Varicosity
D. Edema

B

1532. What is a body tissue called that dies due to lack of blood supply?

A. Infarct
B. Thrombus
C. Embolism
D. Hemorrhage

A

1533. Following a myelogram, what is the fluid that is sent to the laboratory called?

A. CHF
B. CSF
C. CNS
D. BUN

B

1534. What is a tumor called that is NOT cancerous?

A. Malignant
B. Primary
C. Carcinoma
D. Benign

D

1535. The abbreviation "Dx" stands for which of the following?

A. Dissecting
B. Prescription
C. Diagnosis
D. Dictionary

C

1536. The abbreviation "Hx" stands for which of the following?

A. Prognosis
B. History
C. High blood pressure
D. Heart attack

B

1537. Which of the following refers to the abbreviation "IM"?

A. A method of administering a drug
B. The eye
C. A means of locating a patient
D. The leg

A

1538. An abnormal connection between two surfaces is known as what?

A. Diverticulum
B. Polyp
C. Fistula
D. Stricture

C

1539. What is a track from a deep structure (e.g. bone) to the skin called?

A. Fistula
B. Stenosis
C. Lesion
D. Sinus

D

1540. An "NG" tube passes from where to where?

A. Mouth to stomach
B. Nose to greater opening
C. Mouth to colon
D. Nose to stomach

D

1541. Where would an "ET" tube be located?

A. Stomach
B. Esophagus
C. Trachea
D. Intestines

C

1542. What does the suffix "-algia" mean?

A. Study of
B. Cell
C. Disease
D. Pain

D

1543. What does the suffix "-gram" stand for?

A. Record
B. Deficiency
C. Removal
D. Incision

A

1544. Which of the following is the suffix that means "surgical repair'?

A. -therapy
B. -ostomy
C. -plasty
D. -genesis

C

1545. What is another term for fainting?

A. Palsy
B. Dysphagia
C. Myasthenia gravis
D. Syncope

D

1546. What does the root word "phren" mean?

A. To breathe
B. Diaphragm
C. Lung
D. Tonsils

B

1547. Which of the following prefixes means "painful"?

A. Pro
B. Pan
C. Dys
D. Contra

C

1548. What is the meaning of the prefix "poly"?

A. Half
B. Through
C. Above
D. Many

D

1549. Which of the following prefixes means "false"?

A. Epi
B. Pseudo
C. Para
D. Ante

B

1550. Which of the following root words means "spinal cord"?

A. Pont
B. Gli
C. Myel
D. Plex

C

1551. Which of the following root words means "nerve"?

A. Myel
B. Cerebel
C. Dur
D. Neur

D

1552. Which of the following words means "mono"?

A. Nucleus
B. Color
C. One
D. Iron

C

1553. What is it called when a surgeon makes a new connection between segments of an organ or a tube?

A. Deglutition
B. Emulsification
C. Anastomosis
D. Regurgitation

C

1554. Which of the following is the suffix that means "surgical puncture to remove fluid"?

A. -lysis
B. -ectomy
C. -centesis
D. -cele

C

1555. A patient who has an unusually large amount of fluid in his body tissue is suffering from which of these?

A. Cyanosis
B. Diaphoresis
C. Edema
D. Pallor

C

1556. The complete reversal of all abdominal organs (e.g. the stomach is on the right) is known as what?

A. Hirschsprung's disease
B. Malrotation
C. Duplication of the gut
D. Situs inversus

D

1557. A patient whose skin has a bluish tinge due to a lack of oxygen in his blood is suffering from what condition?

A. Cyanosis
B. Diaphoresis
C. Edema
D. Pallor

A

1558. Which of the following prefixes means "below"?

A. Inter
B. Intra
C. Infra
D. Pseudo

C

1559. What is the meaning of the prefix "contra"?

A. Before
B. Through
C. Complete
D. Against

D

CIRCULATORY AND SKELETAL DISEASES

1560. What does the root word "vas" mean?

A. Atrium
B. Heart
C. Vessel
D. Chest

C

1561. Which of the following root words means "vein"?

A. Phleb
B. Valv
C. Cardi
D. Aort

A

1562. Which of the following root words means "blood"?

A. Reticul
B. Hemat
C. Myel
D. Leuk

B

1563. The sudden stoppage of heart action is referred to as what?

A. Cardiac arrest
B. Resuscitation
C. Cyanosis
D. Shock

A

1564. "Heart attack" is a descriptive term for which of the following clinical conditions?

A. Chest pain
B. Rapid heart rate
C. Occluded coronary artery
D. Difficulty breathing

C

1565. A patient has an extra heart sound between normal heart sounds. What is this called?

A. Heart attack
B. Angina
C. Arrhythmia
D. Heart murmur

D

1566. Which of the following is the technical term for a "heart attack"?

A. Angina pectoris
B. Myocardial infarction
C. Dyspnea
D. Palpitations

B

1567. A patient whose blood is lacking in those components that provide the immune response may have what?

A. Mononucleosis
B. Elephantiasis
C. Hodgkin's disease
D. AIDS

D

1568. Which of the following is an acute infectious disease that primarily affects lymphoid tissue?

A. Atherosclerosis
B. Mononucleosis
C. Leukemia
D. Staphylococci

B

1569. The constriction or narrowing of a blood vessel is referred to as what?

A. Aneurysm
B. Edema
C. Thrombosis
D. Stenosis

D

1570. Which of the following diseases is the result of insufficient red blood cells or hemoglobin?

A. Jaundice
B. Cyanosis
C. Phlebitis
D. Anemia

D

1571. Which of the following is the definition for the term "dyspnea"?

A. Excess of fluid in tissues
B. Rapid heartbeat
C. Difficulty breathing
D. Abnormal blood flow

C

1572. Which of the following refers to acute chest pain due to inadequate oxygen supply?

A. Angina pectoris
B. Palpitation
C. Regurgitation
D. Cardiac arrhythmia

A

1573. "Swelling" caused by excessive fluid in the tissues is called what?

A. Edema
B. Anemia
C. Jaundice
D. Cyanosis

A

1574. Which of the following is a serious state of shock resulting from an allergic reaction?

A. Cardiogenic shock
B. Anaphylactic shock
C. Insulin shock
D. Traumatic shock

B

1575. A dilatation or sac-like formation in a weakened blood vessel wall is referred to as what?

A. Embolism
B. Aneurysm
C. Thrombus
D. Phlebo

B

1576. What is the name of the disease that is best known as "hardening of the arteries"?

A. Hypertension
B. Tachycardia
C. Arteriosclerosis
D. Arterial varices

C

1577. Which of the following is the definition of the term "embolism"?

A. Obstruction of a blood vessel
B. High blood pressure
C. Inflammation of a vein
D. Rapid heart rate

A

1578. What does the root word "thromb" mean?

A. Nucleus
B. Protein
C. Round
D. Clot

D

1579. Which of the following root words means "heart"?

A. Steth
B. Cyan
C. Cardi
D. Angi

C

1580. The term "tachycardia" is defined as what?

A. High blood pressure
B. Stopping of the heart
C. Rapid heart rate
D. Inflammation of the heart

C

1581. What is a blood clot called that has formed within a vessel?

A. An infarct
B. A thrombus
C. An embolism
D. A hemorrhage

B

1582. A severe narrowing of the aorta is called what?

A. Aortic transposition
B. Coarctation of the aorta
C. Patent ductus arteriosus
D. Pulmonary stenosis

B

1583. Which of the following root words means "protection"?

A. Thromb
B. Morph
C. Eosin
D. Immun

D

1584. Rapid, irregular, ineffective twitches of the ventricles is referred to as what?

A. Ventricular fibrillation
B. Ventricular arrhythmia
C. Ventricular palpitations
D. Ventricular regurgitation

A

1585. A patient who is lacking the substance in the blood for clotting is suffering from what condition?

A. Aplastic anemia
B. Hemophilia
C. Sickle-cell anemia
D. Leukemia

B

1586. Which of the following refers to a person's heart beating irregularly?

A. Heart attack
B. Angina
C. Arrhythmia
D. Heart murmur

C

1587. What is the meaning of the root word "angi"?

A. Vessel
B. Artery
C. Vein
D. Aorta

A

1588. Which of the following refers to a noticeably rapid heartbeat?

A. Palpitations
B. Angina
C. Cardiac arrest
D. Congenital heart

A

1589. Which of the following is the technical name for high blood pressure?

A. Phlebitis
B. Stenosis
C. Aneurysm
D. Hypertension

D

1590. What is a blue coloration of tissue, due to lack of oxygen, called?

A. Jaundice
B. Leukemia
C. Cyanosis
D. Erythema

C

1591. Leukemia is a disease that results from an unrestrained growth of which type of cell?

A. Red blood cell
B. White blood cell
C. Plasma
D. Erythrocytes

B

1592. Esophageal varices is a condition that is characterized by which of the following?

A. Dilated esophagus
B. Blood clots in the esophagus
C. Varicose veins of the esophagus
D. Small blood supply to the esophagus

C

1593. An inflammation of a vein is known as what?

A. Phlebitis
B. Thrombosis
C. Embolitis
D. Edemitis

A

1594. The condition where the body of L5 slips forward on top of SI is known as what?

A. Annulus fibrosis
B. Slipped disk
C. Spondylolisthesis
D. A compression fracture

C

1595. An infection of the bone is referred to as what?

A. Osteomyelitis
B. Osteoblast
C. Osteosclerosis
D. Osteoporosis

A

1596. Which of the following describes a compound fracture?

A. The broken bone pierces the skin
B. The break is in the lower leg
C. The bone is in many small pieces
D. The fracture is in the skull

A

1597. What is the condition found in older women that involves the gradual loss of calcium from the bones?

A. Osteosarcoma
B. Osteoporosis
C. Achondroplasia
D. Osteogenesis

B

1598. Which of the following is the root word that means "rib"?

A. Orth
B. Rachi
C. Lord
D. Costa

D

1599. Which of the following root words means "bone"?

A. Verte
B. Kypho
C. Oste
D. Orth

C

1600. A failure of the neural arch of a vertebra to close creates the condition known as what?

A. Osteogenesis
B. Spondylolisthesis
C. Slipped disk
D. Spina bifida

D

1601. What type of fracture to the floor of the orbit will result from a direct blow to the eye?

A. Colles' fracture
B. Trimalleolar fracture
C. Blow out fracture
D. Compression fracture

C

1602. What is a fracture at the distal end of the radius called?

A. Colles' fracture
B. Fatigue fracture
C. March fracture
D. Jones fracture

A

1603. What type of fracture is often seen in children where one side of a bone is broken and the other side is bent?

A. Compression fracture
B. Greenstick fracture
C. Colles' fracture
D. Jones fracture

B

1604. When a bone is splintered or crushed into many pieces it is what type of fracture?

A. Compound
B. Comminuted
C. Blow out
D. Impacted

B

1605. When one bone segment is driven into another it is known as what type of fracture?

A. Compound
B. Fatigue
C. Blow out
D. Impacted

D

1606. What does the root word "orth" mean?

A. Straight
S. Vertebra
C. Bone
D. Fracture

A

1607. Which of the following is an inflammation of the fluidfilled sacs that surround a joint?

A. Bursitis
B. Callus
C. Atrophy
D. Acetylcholine

A

1608. Which of the following is a benign bone tumor?

A. Osteogenic sarcoma
B. Osteoma
C. Osteoarthritis
D. Osteodystrophy

B

1609. "Gout" is a disease of the joint that is a result of which of the following?

A. Inactivity
B. Inflammation
C. Injury
D. Excessive uric acid

D

1610. Which of the following is described as a shrinkage or wasting of bone due to inactivity?

A. Callus
B. Sprain
C. Atrophy
D. Bursa

C

1611. "Osteoarthritis" is defined by which of the following?

A. Degenerative muscle disease
B. Chronic joint disease
C. A joint injury
D. Malignant joint tumor

B

1612. Which of the following is a primary bone malignancy?

A. Osteogenic sarcoma
B. Osteoma
C. Rickets
D. Osteomyelitis

A

1613. Which of the following fractures is caused by a diseased bone?

A. Fatigue fracture
B. Pathological fracture
C. Medullary fracture
D. Disuse atrophy fracture

B

DIGESTIVE AND URINARY DISEASES

1614. Hirschsprung's disease involves which of the following?

A. Stomach
B. Small intestine
C. Large intestine
D. Pancreas

C

1615. What is another name for a bowel obstruction?

A. Volvulus
B. Ileus
C. Calculus
D. Diverticulosis

B

1616. What is the name of a growth that extends into a cavity from the mucosal lining, often on a stalk?

A. Diverticulum
B. Polyp
C. Fistula
D. Stricture

B

1617. Which of the following is the medical term for an inflammation of the gallbladder?

A. Cholelithiasis
B. Cholecystitis
C. Choleangiogram
D. Cystitis

B

1618. What is the medical name for a twisting or kinking of the bowel?

A. Ileus
B. Diverticulosis
C. Volvulus
D. Intussusception

C

1619. Hepatitis is a contagious disease that affects which of the following organs?

A. Stomach
B. Gallbladder
C. Pancreas
D. Liver

D

1620. What is it called when part of the bowel telescopes into the adjacent bowel?

A. Diverticulitis
B. Malrotation
C. Ileoscopy
D. Intussusception

D

1621. What is pyloric stenosis?

A. Opening between stomach and duodenum
B. Narrowing of pyloric orifice
C. A gland of the stomach
D. The first part of the pylorus

B

1622. Pyloric stenosis is most often found in which of the following?

A. Young infants
B. Children
C. Young adults
D. Older adults

A

1623. A patient who has gallstones is said to have what condition?

A. Cholelithiasis
B. Cholecystitis
C. Choleangiogram
D. Cystitis

A

1624. A life-threatening condition, when the esophagus ends in a blind pouch, is referred to as what?

A. Esophageal atresia
B. Esophagitis
C. Pyloric stenosis
D. Hiatal hernia

A

1625. What is it called when part of the stomach slips through the diaphragm into the thorax?

A. Esophagitis
B. Hiatal hernia
C. Diaphragmatic weakening
D. Gastric bulge

B

1626. If a patient suffers from dysphagia, they would have difficulty doing which of the following?

A. Eating
B. Swallowing
C. Talking
D. Breathing

B

1627. Which of the following terms refers to swallowing?

A. Deglutition
B. Peristalsis
C. Emulsification
D. Mastication

A

1628. Which of the following conditions best describes an unusually large amount of fluid in the peritoneal cavity?

A. Diverticulosis
B. Ascites
C. Jaundice
D. Cirrhosis

B

1629. Crohn's disease involves which of the following systems or organs?

A. Stomach
B. Intestines
C. Gallbladder
D. Pancreas

B

1630. "Loss of appetite" describes which of the following conditions?

A. Anorexia
B. Enteritis
C. Volvulus
D. Regional ulcers

A

1631. A patient suffering from gastritis has which of the following problems?

A. Twisting of stomach
B. Distended rugae
C. Inflammation of the stomach
D. Ulcers

C

1632. The formation of pouches or sacs in the colon is called what?

A. Diverticulitis
B. Diverticulosis
C, Diverticulum
D. Diverticula

B

1633. What would an ulcer in the stomach or duodenum be called?

1. Gastritis
2. Enteritis
3. Peptic ulcer

A. 1 only
B. 3 only
C. 1 & 2 only
D. 1, 2 & 3

B

1634. What is another name for a "hairball"?

A. Ileus
B. Cholelith
C. Volvulus
D. Bezoar

D

1635. Which of the following describes an inflammation of the abdominal cavity lining?

A. Peritonitis
B. Gastritis
C. Enteritis
D. Diverticulitis

A

1636. What does the root word "nephr" mean?

A. Renal pelvis
B. Kidney
C. Cortex
D. Bladder

B

1637. What is the condition called when a patient's kidneys cannot excrete any urine?

A. Dysuria
B. Anuria
C. Hematuria
D. Polyuria

B

1638. Which of the following root words means "renal pelvis"?

A. Pyel
B. Vesic
C. Trigon
D. Glomerul

A

1639. Which of the following is broken down into the two major categories of "gross" and "microscopic"?

A. Hematuria
B. Cystitis
C. Reflux
D. Hydronephrosis

A

1640. Which of the following is another name for a kidney stone?

A. Pyelonephritis
B. Cystitis
C. Renal calculus
D. Hematuria

C

1641. Which of the following terms describes hematuria?

A. Painful urination
B. Inability to urinate
C. Blood in the urine
D. Frequent urination

C

1642. An obstructed ureter will cause the renal pelvis to dilate with urine. What is this condition called?

A. Incontinence
B. Nephrolithiasis
C. Urenia
D. Hydronephrosis

D

1643. Wilm's tumor involves which of the following?

A. Adrenal gland
B. Bladder
C. Kidney
D. Ureter

C

1644. Which of the following defines dysuria?

A. Painful urination
B. Inability to urinate
C. Frequent urination
D. Constant urination

A

1645. What is an inflammation of the kidney and renal pelvis called?

A. Renalitis
B. Pyelonephritis
C. Cystitis
D. Uritis

B

1646. Which of the following relates to the outer layer of the kidney?

A. Medulla
B. Cortex
C. Glomerulus
D. Urinary

B

1647. Cystitis would be an inflammation of which of the following organs?

A. Kidney
B. Pancreas
C. Urinary bladder
D. Adrenal gland

C

RESPIRATORY AND OTHER DISEASES

1648. What is it called when air enters the pleural space?

A. Pleural effusion
B. Hemothorax
C. Pneumothorax
D. Pneumogram

C

1649. What is it called when part of a patient's left bronchial tree is blocked, causing a partial collapse?

A. Pneumothorax
B. Atelectasis
C. Hemothorax
D. Pleural effusion

B

1650. An upper respiratory disease would be located where?

1. Nose and throat
2. Trachea
3. Bronchi

A. 1 only
B. 2 only
C. 1 & 3 only
D. 2 & 3 only

A

1651. Which of the following means surgically opening the trachea to free the air passageway?

A. Tracheotomy
B. Pharyngeal incision
C. Trachectomy
D. Respiratory removal

A

1652. Which of the following diseases is characterized by a hypersensitivity to various allergens?

A. Influenza
B. Bronchitis
C. Bronchial asthma
D. Emphysema

C

1653. Which of the following diseases is considered contagious?

A. Emphysema
B. Bronchial asthma
C. Bronchitis
D. Tuberculosis

D

1654. A chronic dilatation and distention of the bronchi with subsequent infection is known as what?

A. Bronchioles
B. Bronchiectasis
C. Hemoptysis
D. Abscess

B

1655. Which of the following is an infection of the upper respiratory tract?

A. Atelectasis
B. Bronchitis
C. Influenza
D. Pleurisy

C

1656. The technical name for "lung cancer" is which of the following?

A. Bronchogenic carcinoma
B. Pleural sarcoma
C. Bronchialoma
D. Dyspnea

A

1657. Which of the following is a lower respiratory disease?

A. Tonsillitis
B. Influenza
C. Hay fever
D. Bronchitis

D

1658. Pneumonia is described by which of the following?

A. An acute inflammation of the lung
B. Air in the lungs
C. Lung congestion
D. Collapsed lung

A

1659. Dyspnea is associated with many lung diseases. What is dyspnea?

A. Rapid breathing
B. Irregular respiratory rate
C. Labored or difficult breathing
D. Shallow breathing

C

1660. Which of the following diseases is characterized by an inflammation of the pleural membranes?

A. Consolidation
B. Atelectasis
C. Asthma
D. Pleurisy

D

1661. What is a disease of smokers that is characterized by inflation of the lungs with trapped air in the alveoli?

A. Bronchitis
B. Emphysema
C. Hemoptysis
D. Asthma

B

1662. What is it called when fluid collects in the pleural space?

A. Pleural effusion
B. Hemothorax
C. Pneumothorax
D. Pneumogram

A

1663. A patient with a knife wound to the chest might demonstrate which of the following on his chest radiograph?

1. Pneumothorax
2. Hemothorax
3. Atelectasis

A. 1 & 2 only
B. 1 & 3 only
C. 2 & 3 only
D. 1, 2 & 3

D

1664. Which of the following would describe a hemiplegic?

A. Paralyzed from the waist up
B. Paralyzed from the waist down
C. Paralyzed on one side
D. Paralyzed in all four extremities

C

1665. Which of the following would describe a quadriplegic?

A. Paralyzed from the waist up
B. Paralyzed from the waist down
C. Paralyzed on one side
D. Paralyzed in all four extremities

D

1666. A goiter is associated with which of the following glands?

A. Adrenal
B. Pituitary
C. Thyroid
D. Prostate

C

1667. If a patient had a blocked fallopian tube, which of the following radiographic exams may be performed?

A. Sialogram
B. Hysterosalpingogram
C. Cystourethrogram
D. Fallopioscopy

B

1668. A patient with breast cancer may be faced with which of the following surgical procedures?

A. Mastectomy
B. Lobotomy
C. Laparotomy
D. Thoracotomy

A

1669. What is a pregnancy called that is NOT in the uterus?

A. Endometriosis
B. Eclampsia
C. Ectopic
D. Fibrocystic

C

1670. Which of the following is a very serious inflammation of the brain?

A. Spinalitis
B. Encephalitis
C. Hydrocephalus
D. Meningitis

B

1671. What is it called when a patient's ventricles are filled with a large amount of cerebrospinal fluid?

A. Meningitis
B. Epilepsy
C. Spina bifida
D. Hydrocephalus

D

1672. The disease process involving cancer of the lymphatic system is called what?

A. Mononucleosis
B. Elephantiasis
C. Hodgkin's disease
D. AIDS

C

1673. What is the condition called when tissue dies due to lack of blood supply and then decomposes?

A. Acne
B. Gangrene
C. Eczema
D. Impetigo

B

1674. Diabetes mellitus is a condition caused by lack of insulin secretion from which of the following organs?

A. Stomach
B. Kidneys
C. Pituitary gland
D. Pancreas

D

1675. Which of the following is a malignant tumor of surface epithelial tissue?

A. Sarcoma
B. Carcinoma
C. Osteoma
D. Neoplasm

B

1676. Which of the following tumors is an invasive tumor capable of metastasis and likely to cause death?

A. Benign tumor
B. Malignant tumor
C. Wart
D. Teratoma

B

1677. What does the term "metastasis" mean?

A. Spread of cancer to a distant site
B. A non-malignant tumor
C. A malignant tumor
D. The absence of cancer

A

1678. Which of the following terms describes a tumor and actually means "new growth"?

A. Carcinoma
B. Sarcoma
C. Neoplasm
D. Osteoma

C

1679. Which of the following tumors is a non-malignant tumor?

A. Benign tumor
B. Carcinoma
C. Sarcoma
D. Adenocarcinoma

A

1680. Which of the following is a malignant tumor of connective tissue?

A. Sarcoma
B. Carcinoma
C. Osteoma
D. Neoplasm

A

1681. Which of the following is a chronic degenerative liver disease?

A. Cystic fibrosis
B. Cirrhosis
C. Ascites
D. Cholecystitis

B

1682. Splenomegaly is defined by which of the following?

A. Cancer of the spleen
B. Inflammation of the spleen
C. Absence of the spleen
D. Enlargement of the spleen

D

1683. Hepatitis is an inflammatory disease of which of the following organs?

A. Spleen
B. Gallbladder
C. Pancreas
D. Liver

D

1684. What is a goiter?

A. Enlarged thyroid gland
B. Enlarged pituitary gland
C. Enlarged adrenal gland
D. Enlarged pineal gland

A

1685. Which of the following is a mental and physical retardation due to congenital thyroid deficiency?

A. Addison's disease
B. Cretinism
C. Crohn's disease
D. Acromegaly

B

1686. A patient who has an elevated blood glucose level would be described as being what?

A. Alcoholic
B. Hypoglycemic
C. Hyperglycemic
D. Hypothelmic

C

1687. What is it called when a woman reaches an age when her menstrual cycle stops?

A. Menarche
B. Menorrhagia
C. Metrorrhagia
D. Menopause

D

1688. A common problem among elderly men is prostatic enlargement. Which radiographic exam will show this?

1. IVU
2. Cystogram
3. Voiding cystourethrogram

A. 1 only
B. 1 & 2 only
C. 1 & 3 only
D. 1, 2 & 3

D

1689. A stroke victim may be alert but suffering from aphasia. Which of the following describes this condition?

A. Loss of speech
B. Loss of sight
C. Loss of feeling
D. Loss of taste

A

1690. Which of the following is an injury to the brain caused by a severe impact?

A. Concussion
B. Convulsion
C. Contusion
D. Conversion

A

1691. Which of the following is a disease of abnormal electrical discharges in the brain?

A. Encephalitis
B. Epilepsy
C. Hydrocephalus
D. Meningitis

B

1692. Which of the following conditions usually results in a loss of consciousness?

A. Convulsion
B. Contusion
C. Conflict
D. Concussion

D

1693. An inflammation of the covering of the brain and/or spinal cord is called what?

A. Meningitis
B. Cerebralitis
C. Poliomyelitis
D. Multiple sclerosis

A

1694. Which of the following describes involuntary contractions of voluntary muscles?

A. Convulsions
B. Glioma
C. Hydrocephalus
D. Multiple sclerosis

A

1695. Which of the following is commonly called "skin cancer"?

A. Eczema
B. Psoriasis
C. Epidermitis
D. Squamous cell carcinoma

D

1696. Mongolism is also referred to as which of the following?

A. Turner's syndrome
B. Crohn's disease
C. Down's syndrome
D. Jones disease

C

1697. A disorder that is present at birth is known as what?

A. Mutation
B. Congenital
C. Homogeneous
D. Homozygous

B

1698. Which of the following is a branch of science that deals with the aged?

A. Pediatrics
B. Geriatrics
C. Senility
D. Alzheimers

B

1699. A patient with cataracts has which of the following conditions?

A. Opacity of the eye lens
B. Hormone deficiency
C. Constipation
D. Ulcers

A

1700. An elderly patient who has a loss of mental, physical and emotional control is said to be what?

A. Geriatric
B. Homeostatic
C. Spastic
D. Senile

D

1701. Which of the following diseases involves chronic inflammation of the intestines?

A. Crohn's disease
B. Addison's disease
C. Alcoholism
D. Grave's disease

A

VENIPUNCTURE

1702. The Centers for Disease Control (CDC) recommends that all health care providers:

1. wear gloves when touching blood, body fluids or broken skin of all patients .
2. wash hands immediately if they become contaminated with blood or other body fluids.
3. place syringes, needles and sharp items in puncture - resistant containers for disposal.

A. 1 & 2 only
B. 1 & 3 only
C. 2 & 3 only
D. 1, 2 & 3

D

1703. Which of the following refers to the gauge of a needle?

A. Length of needle, hub to tip
B. Diameter size of needle
C. Size of opening
D. Color of the winged - tip

B

1704. When selecting a venipuncture site, it is preferable to select the most _____ site in which the desired size needle can be accommodated.

A. medial
B. lateral
C. proximal
D. distal

D

1705. When performing an intravenous injection you should first:

A. apply a tourniquet.
B. clean the injection site with an alcohol swab.
C. check the patient's identification.
D. explain the exam to the patient.

C

1706. When performing an intravenous injection, when should the tourniquet be removed?

A. Before the insertion of the needle
B. After the insertion of the needle, before injection
C. After the insertion of the needle, after injection
D. After the needle is removed

B

1707. In practicing universal precautions, when you may be exposed to a patient's blood you should:

A. assume that the patient does not have a communicable disease.
B. avoid that patient.
C. act as if the patient may have a bloodborne disease.
D. ask the patient if he/she is HIV positive.

C

1708. _____ is the escape of fluid from a vessel into the surrounding tissue.

A. Intravenous therapy
B. Extravasation
C. Embolization
D. Enterolysis

B

1709. A (an) _____ most accurately describes a large amount of pharmaceutical preparation that is injected at one time.

A. bolus
B. infusion
C. injection
D. drip

A

1710. A typical flow rate for a drip infusion is:

A. 10 - 20 drops/second.
B. 10 - 20 drops/minute.
C. 30 - 50 drops/minute.
D. 50 - 60 drops/minute.

B

1711. How does a negative contrast agent appear on a radiograph?

A. Less dense than surrounding tissue
B. More dense than surrounding tissue
C. The same density as surrounding tissue
D. More blurred than surrounding tissue

B

1712. Non-ionic water-soluble iodinated contrast media:

A. contains no iodine.
B. produces no adverse reactions.
C. does not dissolve into charged particles.
D. is less expensive than ionic water-soluble contrast media.

C

1713. A water-soluble iodinated contrast media whose osmolality is high:

A. has more particles in solution and results in increased adverse reactions.
B. has more particles in solution and results in decreased adverse reactions.
C. has fewer particles in solution and results in increased adverse reactions.
D. has fewer particles in solution and results in decreased adverse reactions.

A

1714. Allergic reactions to water-soluble iodinated contrast media is thought to be due to the release of _____ by cells in the body.

A. ions
B. hormones
C. adrenalin
D. histamine

D

1715. _____ is the number of particles in a solution per kilogram of water.

A. Permeability
B. Osmolality
C. pH
D. Osmosis

B

1716. When charting drug information, which of the following is NOT necessary?

A. Name of drug
B. Gauge of needle used
C. Route of administration
D. Date and time

B

1717. Medication that is administered sublingually is put:

A. under the tongue.
B. under the skin.
C. in the vein.
D. on the skin.

A

1718. Which of the following reactions to contrast media does NOT usually require treatment?

A. Laryngeal edema
B. Nausea and vomiting
C. Dyspnea
D. Bronchospasm

B

1719. Which of the following may help make veins more prominent on patients whose veins are difficult to locate?

1. Pat or rub the area
2. Apply hot packs
3. Allow arm to hang

A. 1 only
B. 1 & 3 only
C. 2 & 3 only
D. 1, 2 & 3

D

1720. Which of the following patient factors is NOT a consideration for the administration of contrast media?

A. Age
B. Presence of renal disease
C. Gender
D. Presence of hypertension

C

1721. The primary disadvantage of oil-based iodinated contrast media is:

A. its high cost.
B. the high incidence of adverse reactions.
C. its limited availability.
D. that it isn't absorbed in the body.

D

1722. Oil-based iodinated contrast media is commonly used during a(n):

A. sialogram.
B. myelogram.
C. urogram.
D. choleangiogram.

A

1723. A very high creatinine level is:

A. an indication for an UGI.
B. an indication for an IVU.
C. a contraindication for an UGI.
D. a contraindication for an IVU.

D

1724. The preferable water-soluble iodinated contrast media would be:

A. ionic with high osmolality.
B. nonionic with high osmolality.
C. ionic with low osmolality.
D. nonionic with low osmolality.

D

1725. In what order should the following be done to discontinue a contrast media administration?

1. Elevate extremity and apply pressure until all bleeding stops
2. Quickly, smoothly and gently remove cannula from the vein
3. Place sterile gauze over puncture site

A. 1, 2 & then 3
B. 2, 1 & then 3
C. 3, 2 & then 1
D. 3, 1 & then 2

C

1726. After the administration of contrast media, which is true?

1. Do not recap the needle
2. Bend or break the needle before discarding
3. Do not remove a needle from a disposable syringe

A. 1 & 2 only
B. 1 & 3 only
C. 2 & 3 only
D. 1, 2 & 3

B

Corectec's Simulated Registry Examination

This computerized examination follows the latest examination format of the A.R.R.T. and covers the areas of 1) Radiation Protection; 2) Equipment Operation and Quality Control; 3) Image Production and Evaluation; 4) Radiographic Procedures; and 5) Patient Care and Education. The questions on this computerized examination have been carefully prepared to not only review the material, but to reveal your strengths and weaknesses in each of the five content areas.

To Load Corectec's Simulated Registry Examination on Your Hard Drive:

1. Select an IBM or IBM PC compatible computer.
2. Insert the Corectec CD into the CD drive with the printing face up.
3. Click on the **Start** button on your Windows® desktop.
4. Click on **Run** on the Start menu.
5. Type in d:\setup (substitute the correct drive letter of your
6. CD-Rom drive).
7. The install program will begin automatically. Click the **Next** button to accept the copyright statement.
8. Click the **Next** button to install the necessary files on your hard drive (c:).
9. Click **Yes** to create the directory c:\program files\bkexam08.
10. Click on the **Typical** button to install all the files on your hard drive.
11. Click on **Finish** to complete the setup.

To Run Corectec's Simulated Registry Examination:

1. Click on the **Start** button on your Windows® desktop.
2. Point to **Programs** on the **Start** menu.
3. Locate **Radiography Examination** on the pop-up menu.
4. Click on the **Radiography Examination** icon to the right of the pop-up menu.
5. You are ready to begin. Good luck!